Is God Pink?
Dying to Heal

Mary Jo Rapini, LPC
with Mary Harper

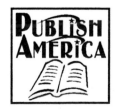

PublishAmerica
Baltimore

First printing

ISBN: 1-4241-5371-9
PUBLISHED BY PUBLISHAMERICA, LLLP
www.publishamerica.com
Baltimore

Printed in the United States of America

Jan, I finished the story for you. You transformed your dying
into an inspiration for how to "really live" each precious day.

Anita – you are blessed,

love
Mary J

Prologue

Alana died within the year. She was a small woman, her face heavily lined from years of working her ranch in the West Texas sun. The uterine cancer that ate away her organs caused her belly to become bloated, yet she rarely complained. She was a stoic, private person. Her guard was up at all times, as if she had been hurt one too many times to allow herself to be vulnerable to anyone or anything. Her life was a sordid trail of betrayal and abandonment by those she loved. She decided one way to prevent this was not to let anyone in. She did not like to talk; Alana saw no need in it.

Most of the time, when I came to see her, she was annoyed. One afternoon I got the courage to ask her if my coming upset her. Expecting a raging "YES," I was quite surprised when she answered "no." She went on to tell me she was angry because she "couldn't go."

"I just lie here and die little by little. I go home, then I come back for more chemo, but I am dying just the same."

She told me about her family, and how her dying was hard on them. She felt that there should be a time when people could just die. I asked her why she thought she couldn't just die. Her answer stunned me, and I will never forget what she said with her sad blue eyes.

"I think that having to suffer is really meant for other people. It's like this, Mary Jo. If I suffer, it's my last act of goodness. I suffer for others."

I was puzzled. Alana was frustrated because I didn't get it. "If you suffer, you allow others one more chance to be kind or compassionate," she explained.

What could I say? There was no answer for that. I reached for her hand and felt her hot, dry hand clasp mine.

Alana looked exhausted. Her lips were dry and cracked, and when she opened her mouth, strings of saliva clung to her yellowed teeth.

"I'm sorry that you have to suffer this way," I said.

"Mary Jo, if you could understand that I'm with God now, you'd be jealous of me."

I didn't understand that before my aneurysm, but I do now. Alana died six days after that visit. It was the longest conversation we ever had. It wasn't much, but it was everything to me.

Chapter One

The Light of God surrounds me;
The Love of God enfolds me.
The Power of God protects me;
The Presence of God watches over me.
Wherever I am, God is!
—Unity Prayer of Protection

I have needed God's protection many times in my life as an ultra marathoner, psychotherapist, lecturer, mother and as number six in a family of nine children. I have always been a risk taker, always pushing myself to run more miles or to achieve more in my professional life, but I never realized how much I would need God's protection that Saturday morning, April 19, 2003.

Since it was Easter weekend and we were planning to have twelve guests for dinner on Sunday, I had a lot to do. I was up early on a beautiful spring morning in Lubbock, Texas. I made the coffee and decided to wait to take my blood pressure pill until after I exercised. I told my husband, Ron, that I would go to the gym for a spinning class and then lift weights. I was happy that Ron was home that weekend. Since November, Ron had been living in Houston, where he is Chairman of Dermatology at M.D. Anderson Cancer Center and the University of Texas Health Science Center. That morning, Ron went out for a haircut while I went to the gym. My daughter,

Brianna, was home from college, and, like her younger sister, Sarina, was still asleep.

Before I left the house, I called my mother-in-law. She had recently been diagnosed with breast cancer. She didn't have much to say. She was in pain from the biopsy and seemed depressed. I remember thinking about her and saying a prayer for her as I drove off to the gym.

The gym was not very popular that morning. People in Lubbock leave town whenever there is a holiday. I was glad, because the spinning class had many bikes available. I found my favorite bike, in a corner where the music was loud and a fan blew cooling air on me. I felt great during the class but did not push myself. After the spinning class, I went over to lift weights on the pec machine. I decided to push myself this time. I was working on my chest muscles. I had a theory that I should be able to lift my body weight with my upper body. I was working up to lifting 106 pounds. Today I was lifting 92 pounds. I did one push, and it hurt so bad that I thought that it would be too hard to do another. I tried one more, though, and heard a loud "POP!"

Something in the back of my neck was out of place. I sat on the machine, afraid to move. I knew that something terribly wrong had happened. Could I have possibly broken my neck?

Chapter Two

I sat frozen on the machine. Something really bad had happened. I couldn't think of what to do, so I stood up. Immediately, blackness began to fill my eyes. I could see only peripherally, and nothing in front of me. Sounds around me became muffled, as if I was under water. It seemed like everything began to move in slow motion. Since I'd fainted in the past, I thought that perhaps I was having some sort of fainting episode. I stumbled over to the water fountain. When I tried to push the lever down, my right leg and right hand started to jerk crazily. I felt weaker by the moment and completely out of control.

Now I was really afraid. I knew that I had some sort of nerve involvement. I was sure that I had broken my neck. I was so weak by now that I slumped down on the floor, right next to the water fountain.

Some guys came over and said, "Hey, Mary Jo! You okay?"

"No, I think I broke my neck!" I told them. "Call an ambulance!"

They thought that I was kidding, but they got down to speak to me. Finally they realized that I was sweating profusely and very ill.

The men ran up to the front desk and got someone from management. They came back with a phone, and a woman started talking to me. I could see her shoes and recognized her voice. It was one of my favorite instructors, and she put her arm around me. She asked me what happened. I told her to call an ambulance, that something bad had happened to me. She called 911 and then called my house. I remember her talking to my daughter Brianna, although I couldn't hear exactly what she was saying.

I started feeling worse, and became very frightened. The right side of my body was numb, I couldn't see very well anymore, I was hot, and I felt very weak. The instructor tried to comfort me by saying several times that I would be okay. She asked for more details of what happened. I didn't have enough energy to tell her.

At this point, I was very aware of my surroundings. I remember smelling the sweaty carpet at the gym, and I could hear all the people talking around me. I tried to push my hair back and realized that it was soaking wet with my sweat. Ron was getting his haircut. I was able to tell them where he was so that they could call him. I could answer all of their questions but was so tired that I didn't want to talk. I began to smell the unmistakable scent of blood and asked the instructor several times if I was bleeding. She kept reassuring me that there was no blood. Actually, I was bleeding, but no one knew it at the time.

Finally, the ambulance arrived at the gym. They carefully loaded me onto the backboard and strapped me down. Just two weeks before my accident, my daughter Sarina had mentioned to me, "Mom, I wonder what it feels like to ride in an ambulance."

"I don't know, and I hope I never have to find out," I'd responded to her.

Now as I rode in the ambulance, I thought about what Sarina had said to me two weeks earlier. Actually, it feels surreal to ride in one. There was a strange relief that I experienced, knowing that I no longer had to be in charge of alerting anyone. They were handling my condition now. I found it easy to submit to these people who were starting IVs and giving me oxygen. They were taking care of me.

My body had a strangeness to it that I didn't understand. It felt like I was in a movie, watching my body from above. Only the pain brought me back into my body. As we headed north on Quaker

Avenue, the bumping and swaying of the ambulance only added to my pain. Each bump of the tires was a further jab that added to the excruciating, stabbing pain in my neck. It was unbearable. I was afraid that I would go mad. I kept begging for pain relief, but due to the nature of the accident and a possible head injury, they were unable to give me any medication. The paramedics kept talking to me and asking annoying questions: "Who is the president?" (I didn't care.) "What year is it?" (Who gives a damn?) "How old are you?" (Should I tell them the truth?)

I just wanted to go to sleep, and they wouldn't let me. They called me by name and kept telling me that we were almost there. They radioed the hospital to say that I was unresponsive. I wanted to say, "No, I'm not, but these guys are annoying the hell out of me." I couldn't say that because it would have taken too much energy.

The next thing I knew, I was in a CAT scan machine at the University Medical Center. The doctors were talking about a lot of blood. There's blood in my head? *My* head? I couldn't believe it, but I was so tired I fell asleep. When I awoke, Ron was by my bed, along with one of my best friends, Becky. She had a baseball cap on and looked like she had just been pulled from her garden. Ron looked scared, and Becky looked like she didn't know what was going on. Ron's expression really scared me, but I felt very safe right then, so was not anxious.

A doctor walked in, and I recognized Dr. Jones right away. He is one of the University Medical Center's finest neurosurgeons. Although Dr. Jones was on vacation that week, he was called into the hospital to see me. He talked to both Ron and me, but most of the conversation was doctor to doctor with Ron. Dr. Jones told him that I had a lot of blood in my head and he suspected an aneurysm. They would need to do an angiogram, and if they found the aneurysm, surgery would be necessary. He explained to me that I might have a weakening in the wall of an artery in my brain that was ballooning with each pulse of my blood. My blood pressure was very high (218/142) at the time of the accident, which added to the danger.

Because it was a holiday weekend, there were no neurosurgeons at the hospital to perform the specialized surgery. He suggested flying me 350 miles to Dallas because they have many neurosurgeons who specialize in the treatment of aneurysms. Dr. Jones told Ron that they would fly me in a private plane, but that he would not be allowed to go with me. He would have to drive six hours or fly on his own. Ron said nothing while thinking about all of this. He was terrified, and he didn't want to let me go alone. He was afraid I would die en route without him.

Ron asked about neurosurgeons at nearby Covenant Hospital. Apparently the neurosurgeon there who operates on aneurysms was out of town until Tuesday. Since it was only Saturday afternoon, it would be a long time to wait. Dr. Jones understood Ron's fear and suggested that we get an angiogram at Covenant, as no one was available to do an angiogram at the medical center. If an aneurysm was found, then perhaps Ron could make a clearer decision. I was transported across the street to Covenant via ambulance. I don't remember much of the ride, just the bumps (which made my head feel like it would explode) and the annoying questions from the paramedics.

I woke up in a cold room in a different hospital. They had just performed my first angiogram, going through the femoral artery with a catheter to look at my brain. I recognized the radiologist who performed it. I had seen him many times before at tumor conferences for the cancer center where I worked. I always thought this doctor to be very kind with cancer patients, and my impression was no different that day. He talked gently to me and told me they didn't see anything abnormal on the cerebral arteriogram, but there was a lot of blood. He asked me how I felt, and I remember telling him my head and neck hurt very bad. From that cold, sterile room I was wheeled on a gurney to the surgical intensive care unit (SICU). Thus began the most sacred part of this journey.

Chapter Three

Easter Sunday, April 20, 2003

I woke up and saw Ron and the girls by my bed. It was about 8:30 a.m. and the second time that I'd been awake that morning. I had gotten up at 5:30 a.m. to clean myself and put on some makeup. I had dried blood all over my hands, and they hadn't washed me very well. I got fixed up because I knew that the girls were coming. I thought that it would make them feel better to see me cleaned up. My face was swollen, but at this point, not terribly so. I looked like I'd just run a long run, because when I run over 50 miles, I also suffer swelling of the face and extremities. I didn't feel very well. I was sick and vomiting, but emotionally, I was not worried or anxious.

The girls smiled and didn't appear to be too worried, but Ron looked very tired and fearful. I started asking Ron about the dinner party that he and the girls were going to have that afternoon. I had arranged it earlier, and I didn't want him to cancel it. Of the twelve people coming, only two knew what had happened to me. Ron was resisting me because he didn't want to have the dinner. He didn't feel like dealing with people. I told him that others would help him, and that he had to tell people what happened anyway. These were all our friends, and it would be our last party before we left Lubbock, as the two girls and I were going to join him in Houston at the end of the school year. I didn't want to disappoint our dinner guests.

In hindsight, I don't know why I was so insistent about that party. Maybe I was thinking that Ron needed their support. I don't know.

I just know that I was adamant that he celebrate Easter with these people, whether I was there or not. Ron asked me if he should call Maria Bravo, who is one of our very good friends. She's a radiologist, and both Ron and I see her as family. She was coming to the party. I knew that Maria would be worried sick when she heard the news, so I told him not to tell her until she got to the party. Ron wanted to call her right then because he knew that she would be very upset. I got up enough energy to actually argue with Ron. The girls smiled because they saw that although I was really sick, I could still hold my own about what I wanted. Ron told me that I was my old stubborn self, but this conversation took a lot of my energy. I was tired again, so I told them to try and celebrate the day and not to worry about me. I reminded Ron how tough I was, and he smiled with an unsure curve to his lips. He would pick up the ham as I insisted, even though the darned ham was the last thing on his mind.

I am a private person, but there was no privacy in that Intensive Care Unit (ICU). I remember hearing the staff laugh and talk loudly outside my door. It struck me how insensitive such behavior is when a person is sick. I reflected on how I had been guilty of doing the same thing outside patients' rooms, and vowed to be more aware in the future.

The ICU at that point was mostly just monitoring me. They still didn't know if I had a bleed from a vein or a more dangerous artery bleed. I was hooked up to an IV, a heart monitor, a blood pressure cuff, and an oxygen monitor. I could still get up to use the portable bedside potty. I heard people moaning in the next room, nurses calling out orders, and family members of other patients crying. Mixed in with the human voices were the sounds of beeping, heart monitors, ventilators, and other unknown machines. The smell of blood and body fluids, alcohol, and other hospital odors was almost overpowering.

It was a struggle because everyone tried to be helpful, but what they didn't understand is that when you are very ill, you're already on another path. You become separate from even your closest friend. I was hearing a voice deep inside me that was keeping me safe and secure. I was not my usual, anxious self. It was odd. My head hurt so bad, and I was throwing up everything, but when people came to visit, I comforted *them*. I'm quite sure that people labeled me as being in denial. "Poor Mary Jo. Maybe she doesn't know how sick she is." Oh, believe me, I knew.

I did what the cancer patients taught me to do. When I asked them how they coped, they said that they submitted to their God because their illness was too big to fight. I remember telling God on Saturday night that I was okay with whatever He gave me. That is a very brave thing to say, and I cannot believe I ever said it. Saying that was what actually freed me and what I believe made me stronger. I submitted to a bigger concept … God … and then I trusted that all would be well. Trusting outside of myself does not come easily to me, but I immediately felt at peace with my decision to submit.

Ron did host the dinner that afternoon, with help from Brianna and Sarina. He wasn't in the mood to have the dinner, but the girls made the most of it. When Ron told everyone about me, some of the guests began crying. Since they are all medical people, they knew how serious my condition was. They knew that I could die at any time.

One of my dearest friends and neighbors, Susan, came to see me Easter afternoon. Because she has five children, she usually celebrates Easter at her own home and therefore was not at the dinner. She brought a card and read it to me since I couldn't see well because of my swollen eyes. She was crying as she told me that many people were already praying for me. I felt so sad for her. I remember telling her that I would be okay. I loved Susan more at that moment than I had loved her over the eight years I had known her. She was so sincere in her grief for me.

Susan is naturally a worrier but now was especially concerned because she's an internist and realized the seriousness of my condition. While Susan is very religious, I never saw myself as religious. However, I am spiritual and have always had the sense that God loves me. She believes that God's love is something we don't deserve but that we receive as a gift, or blessing. I expect God's love and usually get it, although sometimes He uses Tough Love on me. The aneurysm was one of those times.

The closer to death I got, the better the person I became. I thought more about others. I worried less about myself. When I trusted in something greater than myself, I found my true essence. Death has a way of tearing down the facade and making the person more real. The closer I came to death, the more authentic I became. I think about that a lot now. The cancer patients used to tell me that frequently, and now I truly understood what they meant.

I really couldn't eat, but man, was I hungry. I kept craving French fries (salty and fatty), so after the Easter dinner, Ron brought me some of my favorite fries from Arby's. I would eat one or two and barf. Blood came out with the vomit, and it shot out with enough force to hit the wall. When they say projectile vomiting is a symptom of head injuries, they are not kidding.

Ron sent the following e-mail to my family on Easter Sunday: "As you may have heard, Mary Jo is in the hospital with a subarachnoid hemorrhage in her brain. It is not cool to send information like this by e-mail, but it is efficient and is intended to update you without the need for everyone to call. My mother is having breast cancer surgery on Wednesday, so Mary went to add to the situation by aggressively lifting weights (90 pounds or so) on Saturday until she popped a vein in her head and passed out. She was able to get down to the floor so she didn't hit her head on anything. She was unresponsive and went by ambulance to the hospital. Fortunately I happened to be in Lubbock this weekend, even though I am working in Houston. A CAT scan showed 30 to 75 cc of blood around the brain, and an angiogram showed no evidence of an aneurysm, so the exact site of the bleed is not known. She will be in the ICU, and likely will remain there a week, but is still her usual self. Tonight at 8pm she remains the healthiest patient in the ICU, but she still could have bad things happen to her. She has a bad headache but otherwise feels well and has no neurologic deficit. Mary is worried about such things as putting on her makeup and getting curly fries from Arbys. She wants to go home, but cannot because they have to monitor her. She will have a repeat angiogram in a few days. Brianna was here and just flew back to school in Austin tonight. I am staying here in Lubbock with Sarina for now. It is hard to send anything to the ICU, so if you really feel you want to send a card or something, you can send it to our Lubbock address, and I will take it to her. Flowers and all are not good in the ICU. Happy Easter. Love Ron."

Chapter Four

Monday, April 21, 2003
Intensive Care Unit

Early that morning, I woke up to see a very good friend of mine looking at me with a worried expression. An oncologist, he had come to the ICU on his way to work. I was an oncology counselor at the same cancer center, and we had worked together for six years. He was full of questions, but I was tired and too weak to answer them. He seemed concerned that I didn't know how sick I was. I thought he was afraid that I might die and not know it. He knew that I would want to talk about that sort of thing with someone, and I thought that he was testing me to see if I wanted to talk.

I told him that I felt awful, but not as bad as I'd felt after running the 100-mile race in 2000. He laughed, but he looked so sad. His face upset me, and I could see through to what he was thinking. His expression didn't frighten me, but I felt sad. I was sad for him and for everyone who was worrying about me. I don't ever remember feeling sad for myself. Since I think of myself as a selfish person, I remember thinking how unusual it was for me not to feel sorry for myself.

My friend may have felt some guilt, although I'm not really sure. I used to tell him that I got terrible headaches, and everyone who knew me was aware that I was being treated for high blood pressure. They assumed that a thin athlete was probably okay, and he was most likely in denial, too. Everyone, including me, was in shock that something so dangerous could happen to someone who looked so young and healthy.

Friends from the cancer center came in and out all day. Since most of them are physicians and nurses, they didn't have to follow ICU rules about visiting. Many of them had just heard about my accident, and they all wanted to know the details. It was hard for me to talk, and even harder to pay attention to my friends. I listened passively most of the time. It was ironic because active listening is how I make my living. Even at what could have been the end of my life, I still tried but was unable to engage with my visitors. I was just so tired and weak. I felt overwhelmed by the attention. People came in and kissed me, and I had no control over their gestures. I just lay there with a swollen face and eyes, unable to rebuff their advances. They cried, and I couldn't retreat. I was there, a witness to their pain and fear. I kept wishing that I had a bouncer. I needed someone who would guard me from the advances of visitors, doctors, and nurses.

Ron did try to help protect me. Before allowing someone into the room, he tried to decide if a person was close to me or not. Ron was afraid that I would die, and did I need to see these people before I died? I know that it was difficult for Ron, but I was grateful that he turned many of them away, saying that I was sleeping. I was simply too sick to have so many visitors.

Late Monday afternoon, I was moved to a private room. When I got there, the room wasn't ready for me. While we were waiting, the nurse told me about her bad marriage and other personal problems. This comforted me, and I felt more like my old self, like I was doing my job again. I was still very tired, but not as profoundly fatigued as when I was in the ICU. I slept quite a bit that day. They didn't run many tests, and I got my hopes up that I might get to go home pretty soon.

On Tuesday, I had head scans, ultrasounds, blood work, and an MRI. It seemed like I would just get back from one test, only to go for another. I was exhausted. Although I was out of my room frequently, many people came by to see me. I was surprised by how far away from the bed they stood. I must've looked hideous. Perhaps they were frightened by the machines or were overwhelmed by the whole scene. I really didn't have much interest in anyone's conversation. In fact, I didn't care very much about anything.

That night, two of my good friends, Maria Bravo and Gwen Stafford, came up to my room to see me. Maria is a radiologist who is a surrogate mother to me. Gwen knows how to laugh and play. Seeing both of them was a perfect combination for what I needed that night. They mothered, nurtured, and played with me. They didn't look at me with pity. They treated me like I was going to get well. I began to feel better in their presence. I wasn't as tired that night, and those two people made me feel energized. We laughed and talked until about 11:00 p.m. It was wonderful! I felt so content when they left.

Sometime around 1:00 a.m. Wednesday, a nurse woke me up. Apparently my oxygen saturation was low, and I wasn't able to get enough oxygen into my lungs. Normal oxygen saturation is between 95 and 99 percent, and my readings were down in the 80s. I wasn't doing well, and they were concerned. I was moved out of my private room and back into the Intensive Care Unit. They gave me oxygen and began more tests.

I remember seeing Ron's face, and he had tears in his eyes. I didn't know what time it was, but I was guessing that it was early morning. They must have called him in the middle of the night to tell him. He was scared. He talked to me about nothing. He just kept talking, and I was too tired to listen. I had a very strong urge to sleep. I closed my eyes, and he kept waking me. They were afraid that I'd become unconscious or slip into a coma. I didn't care. I just wanted to sleep, and Ron wouldn't let me. I was ANNOYED.

The doctors all gathered around my bed more frequently. I saw them every time I woke up. They were talking in their medical language to Ron. It was Wednesday morning. I was sicker. I was throwing up more and weaker. My head hurt more again. It was the most searing pain that you can imagine. It felt like my head had been run over by a truck. My eyes and face were swollen. My skin was greenish in color. I was lethargic. I was within 24 to 36 hours of death. Ron asked me several times if I was scared. I responded each time, "NO." He kept telling me I was scaring him because I was so calm. I felt secure. I was not afraid, just very tired.

Ron sent this e-mail to friends and family on Wednesday, April 23, 2003: "Mary had a bad day on Wednesday and was put back in to the Intensive Care Unit for monitoring. She is still lucid and neurologically intact, but has a terrible headache and her blood pressure is up. On Thursday she will have a repeat angiogram and if they find an aneurysm this time they will either block it with what they call a coil, or she might even undergo brain surgery. What happens next mainly depends upon what they find on the repeat test. Ron."

Ron stayed with me as much as he could in the ICU on Wednesday night. He made a lot of cell phone calls. He came in and out since cell phones aren't permitted in the unit. I felt worse, and I didn't really care where Ron was or what he was doing or thinking. I felt secure in my heart, but my body was sick.

On Thursday morning, the neurosurgeons woke me up around 6:00. They checked my reflexes and asked me lots of questions to test my ability to understand. I had a terrible headache, and they were very concerned.

The doctors talked to Ron about repeating the angiogram. They explained that the angiogram is an x-ray of the blood vessels in my brain. The doctors would make a small incision in my femoral artery, at the top of my leg. Then they'd guide a small catheter up near my heart, to my aorta, where they'd make a right turn and go up through the carotid artery in my neck. From there, they would snake the catheter into my brain. There they would inject dye into the three main blood vessels in my brain and look for a leak. Ron was told that there's a 1 percent chance that the test itself would cause a stroke, but he signed the papers since he knew that it had to be done. By then, he had brought in the power of attorney papers I had signed many years earlier, never expecting to use them.

They decided to do the angiogram later Thursday morning. If they found an aneurysm, they hoped to place a coil inside of it. They'd detach the coil from a guide wire and add more coils until the aneurysm was packed tightly to stop the leak. The doctors were hoping to avoid brain surgery, since that would be even riskier than the angiogram.

While the doctors and Ron were talking, I saw what looked like a bright light. Their voices faded, and I focused on the large light in the center of my vision. It grew and then took me into it. I remember wondering, "Is this the tunnel?" I was not afraid. I sensed that this was a good thing, and I felt comforted by its gentleness. I felt warm and safe, happy and loved. There were no sounds in this place, just a peaceful silence. The feeling of warmth and love overwhelmed everything else that I could sense.

Soon, I was in an incredible room. There were no floors or walls, but unlimited space. The room was a brilliant white light, tinted with a shade of pink. It felt very soft and nebulous. The light in the room did not move or swirl. Rather, it radiated peace and love to me. While I was in the room, I experienced a feeling of love and acceptance. I felt secure, like being wrapped in a warm blanket.

I felt an incredible force of love. I can't describe it, because there really aren't any words for it. I grew up in a family of nine kids with very loving parents, but I have never felt a human love or acceptance like I did in this room. People have asked me if I felt like it was an endorphin high. I have run 100-mile races, and I've experienced the euphoria of endorphin highs. This was different, because I was in an actual physical place. The room was limitless. I didn't see any walls, but there was a sense that I was in an open, large place.

Someone was holding me, and it felt like God. I didn't see His face, but He communicated with me. I felt like I had been there before, that I knew this place. Now I think about such things as "Why didn't I feel judged?" or "How in the hell did a person like me end up being held by God?" At the time, these things didn't matter, because I felt that God loved and accepted me completely. He was just "God." My humanness limits my ability to imagine all of this now. It sounds as corny or ridiculous to me as it probably does to you. It wasn't, though, and it isn't now. I know with every fiber of my being that I was there in this place with my Creator.

God spoke to me, but not in words as we know them. I could understand, though. His voice came into my being, where I felt His presence and experienced a deep knowingness of His meaning. He told me that He loves me, but that I cannot stay. I began to protest. I was upset! I then demanded, "Why? Why can't I stay?" He told me that I had not loved enough. I took issue with this. I reminded Him that I work at the cancer center, and basically give most of my services away. I told Him that I am on call 24 hours a day, and that I try my best to be present to all of my patients.

"Have you ever loved the way you've been loved here?" He asked.

"No, that's impossible, I'm only a human." I felt childlike, talking to a fatherly presence.

Then I had the sensation that He chuckled and said, "Mary Jo, you can do better. You have to try and give love like you experience here." And then, with the same loving connection and feeling of total acceptance, He let me go.

Although I may have been close to death, certain details stand out very strongly. Ron's voice was very soft, yet clear. And the smell ... all I could smell was blood. I couldn't understand how I could smell the blood in my brain. The other detail I remember is leaving. I left the room, my body, the hospital. I wasn't dead, but I wasn't alive. It sounds odd now, but I was with God. They hadn't given me any morphine or other painkillers, as doctors did not want to mask my mental status. I knew that what I was experiencing wasn't a drug-induced hallucination. This is what happened. Remember that I am a skeptic, and I still have difficulty believing it myself. What my soul experienced I just cannot deny.

Chapter Five

I was feeling very sad, almost grief-stricken. I still felt God's love as I woke up. I was not surprised to be back in the hospital, but I did miss the beautiful pink room. I felt peaceful, but still very sick. It felt like someone was stabbing my head with an ice pick. I was nauseated and just wanted to sleep.

I opened my eyes and felt Ron's hand on my arm, shaking it. He was calling my name. "Mary! Mary! Are you with me?" I worked hard to focus on controlling my pain. I hurt so bad, I was afraid that I'd go mad. "Hold my head off the pillow. My head is so heavy. Ron, would you just hang on to my head?" I was bleeding from my head, down into my neck. All the blood pooled down in my neck, causing excruciating pain. It helped to have Ron lift my head and support it.

Now that I was awake, he told me that I was going to surgery. The doctors were unable to coil my aneurysm and must now do a craniotomy. They would cut open my head and put a clip on the bleeding artery. I realized that Ron was freaking out with this news. His eyes were teary, and he looked so anxious that he couldn't contain it. Normally, Ron is very much in control and reserved. I have seen him like this only one other time in my life, when I miscarried a baby. I was too tired to deal with his emotions. I told him that he had to be strong now, that he needed to get a grip and get control of himself.

In preparation for surgery, Ron started reading all of the written consents that had to be signed. He started to read some damned form to me, and was trying to help me understand what they were going to do in the surgery. He was terrified, and coped by trying to be my legal advisor.

"Do you know that you could be a vegetable?"

"Yes."

Ron started to cry and said, "Mary, you might never run again, okay?"

I heard that, and I took note. I told him, "I will run again. Don't worry."

"You know that you can die?"

"Yes."

I remember saying yes to every question. Most of the questions I didn't really care about, and I realized that we were going through them for Ron to get the damned form finished. He felt like I needed to know what could happen. I was sick. I probably looked like death at that time. It must have been an absurd picture: some guy reading a stupid legal form to a woman who was going to die if she didn't have brain surgery. When people are afraid, they comfort themselves with facts. These were Ron's facts. If he was reading a form and informing me, he felt helpful.

I remember thinking that this was all unnecessary. Ron was unaware that I had been with God.

He didn't understand that I had tried to die and got sent back. I was sure that I would not die in the surgery. Ron was crying, and told me to please come back and not leave him like this. I told him I would be okay. I told him that I talked to God. He had no idea what I was talking about, but thought that I had prayed or something. Ron was so sad. I think that if I could have just explained what had happened to me, it would have made it easier for him, but I was too weak.

The surgery was set for one o'clock in the afternoon of that day, Thursday, April 24. The nurses began to prepare me about 11:00 a.m. I remember hearing them discuss how my head would be shaved. Ron was giving the nurses explicit directions (it was the smallest things that he had control of now). I had always been a big control freak before this experience, but I released the need to be in control during my time as a patient. From the first hospital gown I donned, I knew that I was not in control of my body anymore. That was a scary thought when I was healthy, but it actually was a relief when I became so ill.

The surgery took longer than they expected. The surgeons promised Ron before the operation that they would come and talk to him intermittently. They did not. He was alone. He paced. Below is an e-mail he wrote during my surgery. Most likely it was his way of still feeling useful.

"Mary went to surgery on Thursday at noon. She will have a craniotomy with clipping of an aneurysm they think they see on the latest scan on the middle cerebral artery in the Sylvian fissure between the temporal and frontal lobes. They will shave only half her head and make all incisions in the hair bearing area. It is supposed to be one of the easier areas to access but obviously this is scary stuff. She should be out of surgery by 5 p.m. today, I hope. RR"

As Ron said in the e-mail, the location of the bleed was the Sylvian fissure. It is the area of the brain that affects motor control and emotion. Those are the two areas that most define me. I love to run and to push my body to do more. As a psychotherapist, I find emotions fascinating. My friends say that I'm a very emotional Leo, which I take as a compliment. To live life without feeling would be no life at all. My dear friend Maria Bravo once told me that she believed that the ultimate test is that God takes away our most prized assets and then sees how we grow. Almost losing my most precious gifts, indeed almost my life, was to be a very painful adventure.

It was after 7:00 p.m. when I came out of the surgery. It had been a technically challenging surgery, and they had difficulty waking me up. Ron spent his day pacing, calling people, and talking to God. I asked him later what he thought about while he was waiting. He said that he prayed that my connection to God was as strong as he thought it was. He said that he never prays, because in most areas of spirituality, he is respectful but not sure what he believes. Ron is my closest friend, and the fact that he prayed for my closeness to God was the best thing that any friend could have prayed for.

Why do we pray more when we're afraid or alone? Why does God seem more appealing at these times? Are we programmed to do this, or is it some part of psychological phenomena? Why don't people talk to God or their hearts/souls every day? Are insights less trusted when we are healthy and happy? Maybe our essence or sense of self is exposed more when we are ill or miserable. Maybe suffering is when we peel off that outer layer and realize who we really are. I thought I had suffered and peeled off that layer while running 100-mile races. I was wrong, though. My essence, or sense of self, was realized when I submitted to God's will. That is what became the catalyst for my healing and so much more.

Chapter Six

Ron sent the following mass e-mail at 5:15 a.m. on Friday, April 25, 2003: "Mary did well in her surgery. They found the small aneurysm and clipped it off. Incision is in the hair on the right side. She can move all her arms and legs and talk, though she is exhausted. Still in the ICU. RR"

I woke up that morning about 10:15. Many people had already dropped by and spoken to Ron. I opened my eyes, and Ron was there. His first words to me were, "Hey, Mary, what's up?" I laughed and told him that my head felt like it had been run over. He rejoiced when I laughed because he said that I looked like my old self. He told me that the doctors thought I would be completely normal. Was I before?

I felt very sad hearing him say all of this. Ron confirmed that I would recover, and I realized that I couldn't go back to that space with God. I felt so weak; to live is so much more difficult than being almost dead in that space. I was missing that place I was before the surgery, and wished that I could go back. I was trying to remember everything that happened there. I tried to describe that brilliant pink room to Ron. He thought that I was drugged (I probably was, although I remembered that intense loved feeling). Ron reminded me that I should be so thankful. I was lucky. The type of aneurysm I had carries a 51 percent mortality rate. The doctors thought that I would walk out of the hospital with no lasting injury.

I felt far away. I missed the beautiful pink room and how it felt so peaceful. I had double vision for most of the day. They told me that when the swelling went down, my double vision would go away. My face felt full and tender. I heard things so acutely. Loud voices bothered me. I was sensitive to light, and my sense of smell was heightened. Much to my relief, I did not smell blood anymore.

I was aware that I needed a bath. No one had washed me, and I felt dirty. I felt sticky from dried sweat. I had dried blood on my ears. That blood might have been from several days before, since bed baths are one of the first things to go when you're really sick. I still had to use a bedpan, and I had a urine catheter inserted. They had me sitting in an elevated position in bed. I was totally helpless.

I told Ron that I wanted to get up. Maybe if I moved, I would feel better. He told me that I had to wait until tomorrow to get up. I had a drain in my head that was draining blood. I had a bloody nose, my period, a urine catheter, an IV, heart monitors, and an oxygen monitor. Part of my skull was held together with special plastic strips, which were held in place by titanium screws. Large metal staples held the skin where an eight-inch-long surgical incision had been made from the top of my head to the front of my right ear.

I tried to remember being in that place with God, and fell back asleep. The doctors came to check on me frequently. They kept asking me ridiculous questions.

"Who is the president?"

"Roosevelt."

"What year is it?"

"2004."

"What hospital is this?"

"UMC." I knew that this would get them, as University Medical Center is the chief rival of Covenant Hospital.

The doctors looked at Ron. He said with a grin, "She's playing with you."

I had to laugh. Never again would I ask anyone stupid questions to figure out their mental status. The doctors were pleased with my progress. They were a bit astounded with my wit. They were probably concerned that it might be brain damage masquerading as wit.

This is the e-mail written by Ron about my progress later that Friday morning: "Mary had her aneurysm surgery and did well. She is recovering this am without any neurological deficit. She is said to be in the top 10% after a craniotomy. She ate some eggs and pancakes this morning and is joking with the doctors. She says she feels 100% better. Neck and head pain are much better. She has a slight double vision but that appears to be resolving. She is allowed to sit up in bed but is not allowed out of bed yet. Probably she'll be in the hospital another week, and still is in the SICU right now for monitoring, Ron."

My girls came up to see me on Saturday. My youngest daughter was getting confirmed at church, and I wanted to be there. I asked my neurosurgeon if I could get a pass and then come right back (I had no idea that I couldn't even walk a foot yet without getting weak). He flatly refused. I became very upset. My friend Susan told me that she would go and take pictures. She promised to get them printed as soon as she could. I didn't care about the pictures. I was angry. I told my doctor that even bone marrow patients get passes for special events. He replied, "Mary Jo, you had a craniotomy 48 hours ago. If I let you go, you'd die. You don't understand how weak you are." I was different now. I was not afraid of how sick I was or of dying. My girls, Susan, and Ron left for the confirmation. I felt so alone and depressed.

I flashed back to what cancer patients used to tell me. They frequently said that God talked to them. In the health professions, we say that the patient is experiencing denial or has "too many medications on board." Now I am questioning these frequently made comments. Maybe they *were* talking to God. Maybe they weren't in denial. Perhaps we, the medical profession, are in denial about God. For us to truly listen without judgment and accept the patient's story as his truth might be too scary. Most of us don't like to think of our own mortality. We don't want to entertain the idea that we will ever die, so we try not to listen, or we make excuses for what they say. Did I, as a counselor in the cancer center, respond to the patient with science and logic instead of listening to and validating their experiences?

Chapter Seven

When they moved me to my private room on Saturday morning, I wasn't surprised to see that it looked like a greenhouse. Everyone had brought a plant, as it is no secret that I love flowers. One of the profound lessons I learned when I was sick is that people are more giving. They gave me flowers (at least they didn't wait until I was dead…that's the biggest waste), they prayed for me (believe me, if you live like I do, you should have prayers every day), and they told me that they loved me.

Why don't we tell people that we love them? I have always been puzzled by how hard it is for some people to say "I love you" not only to their spouses but also to family members and friends. Why do we wait until the person is half dead? I know that there are societal implications with this theory. The other person may take it out of context. Saying "I love you" may be perceived as a sexual overture, and we hesitate.

I have family members who are uncomfortable telling me that they love me. I don't understand that. I think that when "I love you" is said and felt sincerely, they are the most healing words in the English language. And if I really love someone, shouldn't he or she know that while alive?

I kept thinking about all of this during my healing. If my assignment is to love more or better, how am I going to achieve that in a society that has rules about bringing flowers to sick or dead people instead of alive and vibrant ones? And if I can say how much

I love you only when you're dead or dying, what about when I really feel like you have touched me and I want to tell you then how much I love you? Who made up these rules?

It was now Sunday, three days since my operation. There was still an increased risk of cerebral vascular spasms, so I was not out of the woods yet. A vascular spasm would not have killed me, but it could have constricted the blood vessels feeding my brain and caused brain damage. I had more CAT scans and ultrasounds. My seven brothers and sisters called me throughout the day. They told me that they were all praying for me. They told me news about what was going on in my home town in northern Wisconsin, and that made me feel more connected. My family was very important to my healing. These are the people who know me best; they had a way of expressing themselves that made me feel whole. Every human heals from the inside out. Medicine tries to convince us otherwise, but the heart and soul take much longer to heal than the body.

My older daughter, Brianna, hates hospitals. The noise, smells, and seeing her mother connected to so many tubes unnerved her even more. When she first saw me with the drainage tube in my head, she ran out of the room. Ron told me later that she threw up. Bri is very sensitive, and seeing me look so different from my normal, athletic self was terrifying to her. I was swollen and weak and couldn't stand up straight. Seeing her mother so vulnerable and fragile didn't fit her view of me. Bri had never needed to take care of me, and I'm sure that she had no idea how to help.

Bri offered to stay with me on Sunday night, even though she was terrified. She had been in Austin, taking her finals, and was home for the weekend. She knew how exhausted her dad was, and felt that she could help by staying with me, which allowed him time to sleep at home. Bri was vigilant with all the nurses and other people coming in and out of my room. She brought me things, trying to make me more comfortable. Bri didn't talk much, but did make me feel like she was there to help support me. I was still her mother, and I did feel the need to protect her. I made light of the staples in my head, the hole in my head where the tube had been (they put a Band-Aid over it), and all of the other uncomfortable things going on with me. Neither of us got much sleep.

I woke up at 4:00 a.m., bound and determined that I was going to go take my shower. I whipped off the oxygen monitor on my finger and started to get up. I was struggling with my IV and my urine catheter, trying to get them into position so that I could stand up when Bri awakened.

"Mom, what are you doing?" she said sleepily.

"Hey, Bri! Help me get out of this bed. I want to take a shower."

"What? No, Mom, that's crazy. I can't help you. You've got too many tubes. I don't know what to do. You might fall. Can't you wait for a nurse to help?"

I took a step while trying to hold on to the IV pole and my catheter. My body began to sway, and I felt like I could fall at any time.

"Bri, if you won't help me, I'll just do it myself. I need a shower."

Brianna knew that I'm very headstrong and that I would indeed take a shower, even if I had to do it alone. Bri got up quickly and cried, "No! No! You get back to bed right now." She panicked, fearful that I would fall. This was my fourth day postoperative, and I could barely walk without holding on to something.

"Bri, you've got to help me because I need to be clean. I'm going to get a cup of coffee and enjoy the sun coming up."

Bri took me by the arms and said, "Mom, listen to me. I feel like I'm going to freak out if you fall or anything, so you have to get back to bed."

"Now Bri. *You* listen to me. I'm your mother. I am getting in that damned shower whether you help me or not. You don't need to help me if it scares you, but just call the nurse if I fall. I *am* taking a shower."

Bri reluctantly helped me to the shower. I'm sure that she was anxious because I had tubes attached and she didn't know how to help. She was afraid that I would fall and really get hurt. I was so dizzy that all I could think of was "Okay, you cannot fall." I didn't want to traumatize Bri any further. It was very difficult to stand in the shower, feeling dizzy and sick. But the cleansing power of the warm water was very healing and made me feel much better. Bri helped to hold me up so that I could dry off, but balked when I wanted help putting on my makeup.

"Mom, nobody cares if you have makeup on."

"But I do. The doctors will be here early this morning, and I want to show them how well I'm doing. I want to go home."

Bri rolled her eyes and handed me my makeup bag.

Chapter Eight

Tuesday, April 29, 2003. One of my closest friends, who now lives in New York, happened to be in town on business. Dianna stayed with me on Tuesday night, and I was so happy to have her company. She brought me a lovely nightgown, which I quickly changed into. I had been wearing a hospital gown until Ron brought me an ugly pair of pajamas. Even though it was a small thing, changing into the nightgown made me feel more like myself.

Dianna and I talked about old times, while she watched my medication schedule and monitored my IV all night. We stayed up late talking. She kept telling me that I would get better fast, and I really think that helped. I told her about the surgery and the weird sensations that I was having. Dianna believes in things that you can't see. Even though she is a physician, she has a belief that science can explain only so much. She was open to my experience with God, and this comforted me.

Dianna and I woke up at 4:00 a.m. Wednesday so that she could fly back to New York. I was sorry that she had to leave, but for two weeks afterward, she called me every day and checked on me. I was touched by her concern, and felt so loved.

Ron sat with me all Wednesday morning and looked like he had aged ten years. Sometimes we forget about the caretaker when someone gets sick. The person who is sick gets all the attention, but being the caretaker is probably more difficult then being ill. You basically have to watch someone you love go through pain and misery, and you have no control over stopping it. Many times, as in my case, the caretaker has to make life-and-death decisions, with no chance to ask the patient how she feels about it. The patient is in another place, and too sick to make decisions for herself.

Ron was scheduled to fly back to Houston that afternoon. He was nervous about leaving. He had friends who were going to assume my care, but he was scared. Ron is a physician, and he knows *everything* that can go wrong. I think that he worried about every possible complication. He knew that if something happened, he would be too far away to get to me in time.

My aneurysm allowed me to see little things so much clearer, such as the love of my friends. Susan arrived that evening and spent the night with me. When you're sick, these gestures mean so much. She brought scones for breakfast, and I will never forget how good those tasted. As she was leaving Thursday morning, I told her that I was getting out of the hospital by Friday, even if I had to go against medical advice.

Susan is an internist and told me that that wasn't a good idea, which is what I expected her to say. I followed that by telling her about my new exercise plan. I was going to walk one mile in the morning and one at night. Susan is my neighbor, so I pleaded with her to walk with me. I was too unstable to go alone. She knew that since I couldn't even walk down the hall on Thursday, there was no way that I could go home on Friday and walk two miles. Knowing me, and how I needed an exercise plan, Susan told me something that I will always remember. She said that when I was ready to walk, she would come and walk with me. Susan said that even if I started out and needed to turn around, we could do that. Susan did what a good friend does when the other is down. She knew that I needed to think that I could do it, and I loved her for that.

Just as I planned, I left the hospital on Friday, May 2, 2003. Ron had previously left me with a bag of clothes. I had asked him to bring me something sexy to wear home and not to forget my heels. (I love heels, and at 5 feet, 2 inches tall, I have always worn them. I could run in them!) I trusted that he would bring me some nice clothes. I was so weak that I never did get around to checking the bag. I wanted to be dressed by 5:30 a.m. so that I could meet the neurosurgeons with my street clothes on and be ready to go.

I opened the bag and found a pair of running pants that had paint on them, an old Wisconsin Badger sweatshirt, and a pair of running shoes. I was livid. I wanted to look like my old self, not some street person.

I called Ron in Houston. No answer. Finally I reached him at work. He was trying to get an early start on his day since he was planning on returning to Lubbock that evening. I scolded him for bringing me those ugly clothes. He tried to be gentle and not tell me how fragile I was. He didn't want to tell me that I would not be able to walk in the heels, that I might fall. He didn't tell me that my walking gait was lopsided. He just let me vent, and said, "Mary, you are not ready for sexy clothes and heels." I was angry. I wanted out of the hospital. I wanted my old self back.

I have two good friends who helped me escape from that place. The hospital felt like a prison to me, and I couldn't wait to break free. My accomplices were Nancy and Evé. Evé is the director of the cancer center, and I worked with him for six years. He was the first to check on me, and I told him that I was leaving the hospital. He looked at me with my running shoes and my old Badger sweatshirt on and tried to hide a smirk. "Are you sure that you are ready?"

"Yes!"

"Aren't you going to be exhausted at home? Here you have all of these nurses who are taking care of you, and at home you'll be alone. Right now you're just lying in the bed, but once you're home and moving around, you'll be really tired."

"Forget about it, Evé. I am going home."

I was irritated at him for even questioning me. Couldn't he see that the hospital had become constricting for me? I listened to him half-heartedly. If he thought for a minute that he could change my mind, he was *wrong*.

My neurosurgeon arrived in the room and examined me yet again. He decided to discharge me and said, "You should go straight to Vegas."

"Why?" I asked.

"Because you are so damned lucky to be walking out of here that I have some money I'd like you to place a bet with!"

I didn't feel lucky, as I knew that I'd have an uphill battle just getting my strength back, and being with God was a lot more beautiful than what I was facing now. (Only later did I learn that the aneurysm I suffered has a 51 percent fatality rate. Of those who survive a subarachnoid hemorrhage, over 50 percent have problems with memory or depression. Most patients experience medical complications, which are often severe in nature. I was indeed fortunate not to suffer any of those complications.)

The doctor wrote out all the prescriptions for me to take upon discharge. Evé saw that I was very tired, and offered to go to the pharmacy for me. I was grateful, as I couldn't think very clearly and was so tired that I couldn't walk more than ten feet without feeling weak and faint.

I called my friend Nancy to tell her that I was leaving the hospital. She arrived about twenty minutes later and said that she would take me home. Evé came back with a big bag of medicine. It reminded me of a trick-or-treat bag full of candy. The full bag shocked me. I couldn't believe that I would need so many medications. I wondered if cancer patients feel overwhelmed with all of their new medications when they go home. Do they feel as scared as I did?

While I was packing up my room, a nurse came in and told me that before I could leave, she would have to take the staples out of my scalp. I was nervous about that, as I'd never had staples removed before, and she was holding a pair of wire cutters.

"Will it hurt?"

"Just a little," she said. (Why do nurses lie like that?)

Nancy jumped up on the bed and held my head like a sister or mother would. The nurse began clipping the staples, and it did hurt.

I was aware that Evé was still in the room, and I could feel his wincing as the nurse clipped the staples.

I felt comforted by Nancy holding me, and was glad that she was there. Although Nancy is a native of Peru and I'm from Wisconsin, everyone thinks that we are sisters. We have similar height and weight, and we have the same color hair and green eyes. Before the accident, I used to see her once in a while because our daughters are good friends. When I had the aneurysm, she came to see me every day and took care of Sarina. Nancy never asked what she could do; she just did it.

Nancy pushed my wheelchair down to the hospital entrance. I resisted using the wheelchair only a little, as I was already exhausted. I had my bag of prescriptions on my lap as Nancy pushed me through the halls. I felt like I was running away...free, but different from the person I used to be.

I left the hospital shortly after noon. I was so happy to see the sun and to feel the Lubbock wind again. It was eight days after my craniotomy. The ride home was only three miles, but the motion of the car hurt my head. It was still hard to hold my head up, and my neck was very sore. My head leaned toward my right shoulder, making it difficult to see out the car window.

I noticed that all the trees had bloomed and that everything was greener, the sky was bluer, and things were much brighter than I had ever seen them. By the time I got home, I was exhausted. Nancy helped me into the house and tucked me into bed. She put her phone number on my bedside table with the phone. (I still keep Nancy's number by my bed, as it makes me remember this time.) Nancy asked me a thousand times if I was okay. I reassured her that I just needed to be in my own home, by myself. The minute Nancy left, I had the urge to jump out of bed. I wanted to walk around the house and see who I was now, but I realized that I couldn't just hop out of bed the way I normally would. I felt very dizzy, so I slowly pulled myself up by the headboard and eased out of bed. I walked unsteadily, holding onto furniture and walls as I made my way around the house. I noticed that the kitchen was a big mess. Ron had brought home plants from the hospital and left them all over the counters. Papers and dishes were piled up. But I wasn't angry. I knew that he was trying to balance taking care of me and working in Houston. Housework could wait.

I looked out the back door into the yard and said to myself, "Oh my God, it's spring here." Everything looked so different. Who am I now? I tried to remember who I was before this all happened. It was odd. Nothing was the same. I wasn't the same. Feeling exhausted, I stumbled to the living room and carefully lowered myself onto the sofa. I could see the new green leaves of the trees in the back yard and hear the wind chime tinkling in the Lubbock wind. I felt the sun's warmth, and relaxed in the peaceful quiet. It wasn't long before I fell fast asleep.

Chapter Nine

The next two weeks of my recovery were filled with pain, reflection, and good friends. Ron came home from Houston to spend that first weekend with me. I was still very weak. Walking was quite a challenge. My head was cocked to my right side, and I couldn't straighten my neck. It was very painful every time I tried to bring my head up to a normal position. I think that the doctors might have injured my neck during surgery. My head had been screwed down, braced to a board to prevent any movement. Most likely my head was turned on the left side so that they could drill through the right side of the skull.

I had terrible headaches on and off throughout the day, although they were worse at night. The headaches felt like pressure inside my head. Sometimes I felt like my head would explode. I was grateful that it was not the same stabbing pain that I experienced with the aneurysm. The doctors never knew what caused them, but said that if they continued, I would need a shunt to get rid of the extra fluid in my brain. I think that this scared the headaches away. In any event, I quit talking about them.

I felt dizzy most of the time. It was not the type of dizziness of the room spinning; rather, I felt that I might black out and faint at any time. My blood pressure was very low as I was taking new medications to try and control it. I could walk from room to room, but had to sit down immediately. I often fell asleep after flopping down on the chair, simply exhausted by the effort of crossing the room. I must have looked like an alien as I walked slowly, trying to hold up my half-shaved head with the bright red staple scars.

My very first walk outside was the Sunday morning after I got home from the hospital. Ron, who was trying to fatten me up, had gone to McDonald's to get me an Egg McMuffin. Dressed in my pajamas with a blanket around my shoulders, I asked Sarina to walk with me to the mailbox. She sensed my weakness and realized that taking this short walk overwhelmed me. Sarina held my hand as I walked shakily down the sidewalk to the curb. I must have been quite a sight, dressed in my pajamas with a blanket around my shoulders, walking slowly with my head leaning to the right. By the time I got back to the house, I was exhilarated, but exhausted.

"Thanks, Sarina. I really needed your help."

"Don't worry, Mom. You look weird today, but it won't be like this forever. Remember, you ran 100 miles!"

Those words made me feel so strong and empowered. What others say when you are healing is so important. I was too weak to think these thoughts for myself. I needed others to validate my situation, and be able to see the big picture. When you are sick, you cannot see the big picture, only your immediate situation. And for me at that moment, my vision was very limited.

Ron was vigilant about watching me. If I even sighed, he would look at me with concern and say rather frantically, "What's the matter?" I found myself becoming irritated by this, but he looked so anxious that I couldn't tell him to cut it out. I did tell him that he freaked me out when he monitored every breath. When he left for Houston on Monday morning, we had a tearful good-bye. He was still worried that something would happen to me, but I was almost relieved when he left. His constant attention was making me feel suffocated.

Since Ron was in Houston on the weekdays, I asked my friends Susan and Erma to spend the night with me. I was afraid that I would die at night and Sarina would find me. I'm all for psychotherapists making money, but not from my kid finding her mother dead in the morning.

Susan and Erma alternated nights sleeping with me. I was on medication to reduce the chance of having spasms in the arteries of my brain. It was very important that I take the pills every four hours. Susan and Erma woke me up when it was time for the medicine. Having them stay with me was so healing. Susan would bring us muffins for the morning. Erma gave me massages at night and kept telling me that I would get my muscle tone back. Little things like that meant so much to me.

Even though I was exhausted, I fought sleep. I just wanted to get back to my normal self. The phone rang constantly with people calling to check on me. Susan came over and did the laundry. Friends and neighbors dropped by to bring food and to visit. I was glad to see them, but after they left, I would fall into a deep sleep. It took so much energy just to talk to my friends.

By Tuesday, I was feeling trapped at home. I hadn't been out since leaving the hospital five days earlier. Riding in a car was difficult because I couldn't hold my head up and the bumps in the road made my head ache worse. Walking still took a tremendous amount of energy that left me feeling very weak. I had never felt so weak and vulnerable. I'd always thought of myself as being strong and able to cope with anything. I was frustrated and depressed.

My close friend and mentor from the cancer center, Dr. Evérardo (Evé) Cobos, came by the house Tuesday morning to check on me. I had not seen him since I'd left the hospital.

"Your hair is growing back, Mary Jo," he commented. "You look much better."

"Thanks, Evé, but I'm just so depressed sitting around the house. I hate feeling so weak."

"What will make you feel better? Can I do something for you?"

"Evé, how about taking me for a ride in my Miata?" I love my car and thought that maybe if I was in my own car, I might feel like my old self again.

"Mary Jo, are you sure you can handle it?" Evé asked nervously. "Maybe it will be too bumpy for you."

"I don't know, Evé, but I think that it will help."

I laugh now when I remember watching this 6-foot, 3-inch man squeezing into my little red sports car. He was a good friend, though, and when you are someone's friend you never know what will be required. I'm sure that this was not as great a thrill for Evé as it was for me.

Evé turned on the CD player, and I was pleased to hear the same music that I'd listened to the day of my aneurysm. While Evé talked about the cancer center, I rolled my window down and just enjoyed his chatting and the wind on my face. I felt like my old, healthy self for a short while. The car was low to the ground, and each bump hurt my head. I tried to hold my head with my hands, but it didn't help much. I didn't want to complain about the pain since I would never admit to Evé that he was right.

Evé drove us down by the cancer center, where we stopped at a red light. As we sat at the light, a white hearse drove right in front of us. It was surreal for a moment. I looked at Evé, and he looked at me. Neither of us said a word. We just looked at each other. Whoever doesn't believe that you can see the soul of a human through his eyes should have been there, in my Miata. I saw Evé's soul, and I am quite sure that he saw mine. I felt so vulnerable at that moment. Evé saw the sadness in my face; I couldn't hide it. I felt almost sad that I had lived. I missed that feeling of being so close to God.

After several long moments, Evé said, "You were really lucky, Mary Jo. You dodged a bullet."

When he said that, I became angry. So many people have told me that I was lucky.

"No, I wasn't lucky. To be lucky would have been to stay with God. We have it all wrong, Evé. We think dying is the worst thing, but I think recovering from all of this and 'being me' now after the aneurysm is much harder."

Evé didn't understand my outburst, and looked uncomfortable. "I'd better take you back home. I have to go back to work, and you look tired."

I was tired, I was depressed, and I was already overwhelmed with my fifth day of recovery. When we returned home, I said good-bye to Evé and immediately collapsed on the sofa. That ten-mile ride had totally exhausted me.

I went to sleep around 1:00 p.m. and woke up at 5:30 p.m. to find Sarina sitting on the sofa with me, doing her homework. Sarina spent most of those days doing her homework right next to me. My good friend Nancy would bring Sarina home from school every day. Sarina and I sat together and talked about school and all of her activities. She did the talking, while I mostly listened.

For dinner, Sarina would warm up food given by my friends and neighbors. She ate, and although I pushed food around, I wasn't very hungry. She was so excited about graduating from junior high school that she didn't seem to notice my lack of appetite. She knew that I was really sick, though, and made allowances for my slow walking. Sarina held my hand and reassured me that I would be back to my old self soon.

Normally, I move very quickly and love to run. Now, though, the constant fatigue and exhaustion were emotionally and physically draining. I knew that if only I could start walking more, I'd feel better. Early in the morning of the second Sunday I was home from the hospital, I woke up and decided to go for a walk. I took my blood pressure medication along with a second blood pressure medicine that had just been prescribed. I was ready to go outside when Ron woke up.

"Hey, Ron, I'm going out for a walk."

"Oh no, Mary, you can't go out by yourself."

"Okay, but I want to go right now. I don't need to change."

"Mary, you have your pajamas on. Why don't you put some warmer clothes on?"

"Ron, I have my flannel pj's on, and they're real comfortable. Besides, nobody will see me at 6:00 a.m." I didn't want to admit that I was too weak to change into other clothes. My energy was so limited that I could have changed or walked, but not both.

"Mary, I really think that you should change."

"I'll put a sweater on. That'll be warm enough."

We went outside and started down the street. We walked about three-quarters of a mile when I started seeing everything turn darker.

I grabbed Ron and said, "I think I'm passing out."

He stopped and lowered me to the curb. I could see the fear on his face. "Mary, what medicine did you take? Are you okay?"

"I took my usual medicine and then that new one."

"I think it's just your medicine. I don't think that you're having another bleed," he reassured me.

I felt very weak and nauseated. I began to get scared that I was having another aneurysm, although my head didn't hurt. I lay on the curb for a few minutes, and then Ron helped me up. I used him as a crutch to get home.

It shook up both of us. It was a psychological setback for me because I wasn't sure that I could trust my body to walk again. Ron was upset because he thought that the medication wasn't appropriate for me. We called my doctor, who told us that it was most likely the new medicine that caused my collapse. I have a low resting heart rate (because I'm a runner, my normal heart rate is about 48 beats per minute). The second medication works to lower blood pressure by lowering the heart rate. The combination of low heart rate and low blood pressure made me feel sick for the rest of the morning. I was very weak, nauseated, and fatigued. Needless to say, I stopped taking the new medicine.

Monday was a new day. Susan came over, and Ron told her what happened. This did not deter Susan. She reassured Ron that she would be careful, but that she knew that it was important for my well-being to keep walking. Ron really didn't want me to walk for the rest of the week, but he could tell that I was determined. I walked one mile that morning with Susan, and by mid-week, I'd added a mile in the afternoon. I still had to walk slowly, with a weird gait, but I did it.

I insisted on walking a mile every morning and evening. Susan walked with me in the morning, and my friend Maria Bravo accompanied me in the evening. If I felt faint, they would just tell me to slow down and they would take my hand. Maria kept telling me how great I was doing, and this really encouraged me and made me feel stronger.

Ron left for Houston on Tuesday of that week. I can only imagine now how difficult it must have been for him. It was an unspoken fear that he might never see me again. I insisted that he go back to Houston, as he drove me nuts with his overprotective manner. I understood him, but found him very frustrating. I was too weak and sick to fight Ron, though, and my heart understood how he felt. His intentions were due to love and fear, but it made me feel so smothered.

My first follow-up appointment with my neurosurgeon was May 8, 2003. My friend Nancy drove me to the appointment since I was still not allowed to drive. When I arrived, the nurses, physician assistant, and neurosurgeon treated me like I was a celebrity. They don't always have good outcomes with brain aneurysms, and they were feeling proud of their accomplishment (seeing me in such good condition).

My neurosurgeon explained everything he did during the surgery: how he had cut my skull open and soaked it in antibiotic solution; how he had performed the surgery and closed my brain with plastic strips, titanium screws, and staples. He explained that I would forever have a titanium clip on the artery in my brain. He also talked about how he put a piece of muslin over a small, weakened area next to the artery with the clip. He informed me that this is often performed, and when it scars over with scar tissue, it actually makes a strong reinforcement for the artery. He went on to talk about the sensations I might experience in the next couple of months (this would be due to the nerves' reconnecting). He said I might feel twinges or zings that were somewhat unusual. I did experience a few of these strange sensations for up to three months after surgery.

Then I asked a very important question: "When could I have sex again?" It was the answer he gave me that made me respect him even more than I did already. He told me that physically, I could have sex now, but he warned me that my husband might not feel comfortable with sex for a while. I was perplexed and asked him to explain this to me. He went on to say that my husband had seen me come close to death. He had seen me with a tube in my head, staples holding my skull together, and throwing up. He said my husband would need time to heal from this sight, and he may be scared about hurting me. I had been thinking of my own needs and not my husband's.

I was so impressed by the way the neurosurgeon explained this to me. He was not uncomfortable discussing sex (many physicians are very uncomfortable talking about sex to their patients), and he didn't turn red, look down, or act fidgety. He addressed the issue very professionally, which is saying a lot, because he knew I was a sex therapist. He understood how important sexuality was to my sense of healing, and he understood that it was important to my quality of life. I will forever be grateful to him for the way he discussed this.

Chapter Ten

It now seems more than just a coincidence that while I was recovering from a life-changing (and life-threatening) event, I had to say goodbye to my life in Lubbock and begin a new one in Houston. My life would never be the same after my experience with God. I had to cope with leaving some very close friends and deal with the uncertainties of life in Houston. Even though we'd lived in Houston before our move to Lubbock, coping with the move and settling into a new house while I was ill was overwhelming.

The movers came to pack us on Friday, the 16th of May. Ron was still in Houston and arrived later that night. Brianna helped me with the movers and directed them so that I could rest. I was still extremely tired and took frequent naps. Whenever I lay down for more than an hour, I got painful headaches. The doctors told me that the headaches were due to postsurgery swelling. The extra fluids in my brain caused increased pressure. I used to wonder if this would be how I would live for the rest of my life, but I tried not to focus on any of the negative possibilities. I kept reminding myself that healing was a process, and that I must trust my body. This was something new for me, as I used to get very anxious about my health. I came out of this whole ordeal trusting God completely. In fact, my increase in faith has been my greatest blessing from all of this. I know now that there is a God, and that He is always doing what is in my best interest.

The movers left late Friday night and returned on Monday to load our things into the truck. This was an all-day event, and Ron worked as hard as the movers. I rested outside on a lawn chair and tried to read. I couldn't read very well because my attention span was short and I tired so easily. Mostly, I slept in the chaise lounge. My next-door neighbors, Susan and David, let us use their RV. It was very comfortable, and Susan reassured me that this would give me privacy. Since they have five kids, Susan knew that the noise would hurt my head. I was so grateful to Susan for lending us her RV. We were able to sleep in there at night and could all be together. Our house was basically empty now, and cold (it is cold in Lubbock in May). It also allowed us to stay close to our home and made it easier for Ron to finish up some last-minute chores around the house.

Sarina stayed with friends as she was planning her graduation from junior high. Brianna was finishing her final exams at the University of Texas and was unable to come home. I was still so weak that seeing friends or thinking about any event was too overwhelming for me. I couldn't really prepare for leaving Lubbock, and much of the time, I rested. This was a stressful time for Ron as he was basically taking care of everything regarding the move and Sarina. My goal was to stay strong enough for the long car trip to Houston.

I did attend Sarina's graduation, which took place the day before we left Lubbock. I wore a newsboy cap over my head, and except for my weight loss and pale color, I looked pretty much like my old self. I was exhausted at the ceremony. I took my pillow along, as my head and shoulders were still achy, but at least I made it. I must have been a strange sight, but everyone there knew about my illness. Many stopped by to talk and told me that they were glad I made it. I was happy to be there for Sarina, but so tired.

Early on the morning of May 21, 2003, Ron packed the car and loaded our two big dogs into the back seat. Sarina stayed with her friends and planned to fly to Houston the following weekend. I was sad to leave Lubbock, and it was hard to say good-bye to our wonderful neighbors.

The trip was long and arduous. Ron stopped every three hours and let the dogs go to the bathroom. My head ached terribly just from holding it up that long. Every bump in the road increased the pain. I tried to lie on a pillow, but there was no comfortable position. We made the trip in one day, driving 572 miles over the Texas countryside.

During the drive, Ron made several calls to the neurosurgeon in Houston to set up appointments for me. There was some question as to whether I had too much fluid in my head, and that had to be assessed. I was a little concerned, but already knew that no matter what the doctor said, I was not going to get a shunt (which is what they suggested earlier in Lubbock). I told Ron that if I could just run, I was sure that everything would heal and be okay. I know it sounds odd now, but that is how much faith I had (and still have) in physical conditioning.

We finally arrived in Houston about 5:30 p.m. Since the movers hadn't arrived, we stayed at Ron's temporary apartment the first night. Ron took me to our new house the next day. I was supposed to greet the movers and tell them where to take the stuff. I was unable to go up the stairs, so I directed them by showing maps of the rooms. Old friends from the first time we lived in Houston stopped by, bringing me food and visiting while the movers unpacked the truck.

Ron came home at lunchtime to check on me. I was exhausted. I was so relieved when he came home early that afternoon. Since our bed wasn't unloaded, I camped out on the floor and slept for the rest of the night.

Sarina came home the following weekend. She became my constant companion. She did almost all of the unpacking, as Ron was still trying to catch up from work not done because of my illness. I was just too weak. I was still unable to lift anything, or walk much beyond a block without resting.

I met my new neurosurgeon May 29 in Houston. I wasn't sure what to expect, but I did know that I was going to decline any further surgery. My Lubbock doctor had discussed the possibility that I might need a shunt to drain the extra fluid, but I had no desire to have a second operation. I was afraid that he might insist that I have the shunt.

"Hello. My name is Dr. Smith." He looked at both Ron and me, trying to decide which one of us was the patient. Ron looked more like the patient. He was exhausted, and his eyes showed the tension of the past few weeks.

"You look great!" Dr. Smith said to me. "Can you walk on your toes?"

As usual, I wore my high heels. It was rather awkward, but I demonstrated my ability to walk on my toes.

"Can you touch your nose? Okay, that's good. By the looks of your chart and films, it looks like you were very lucky. It's really hard to believe that you've had surgery. You're healing much faster than most of our patients," said Dr. Smith.

"When can I run again?" I asked.

"We don't really know the answer to that. We don't see many people like you."

"Well, can I lift weights?"

"We don't really know, because we don't see many people like you."

"Can I ever race again?"

"We don't really know. Once again, there are not enough people like you."

"How high can my blood pressure get before I should be concerned?"

"Well … uh, we really don't know the answer to that either," Dr. Smith stammered.

"Thank you, Doctor. What should I do for follow-up care?"

"Well, be careful, and in one year, we will repeat your angiogram."

As we were leaving the office, I asked Ron, "Why does he say to be careful? What does that mean to a patient when a doctor says 'be careful'? Does that mean that I should live, but don't live too hard?"

"Mary, no one can tell you what to do, because there aren't many patients like you to compare to. Just be careful … quit pushing yourself," he advised.

I reflected on our conversation a lot. That is when I made a conscious decision for myself. I decided that I would live the way that I had been too afraid to live in the past. I would take more risks, laugh more, and try new things instead of worrying about whether or not I was good at it. I began to see myself as having fewer limits. I felt open to new projects that I would never have taken on before my aneurysm. Most important, I quit worrying about my health. I had survived a near-fatal bleed in my brain. I realized that I was strong enough to live with whatever God gave me. Since I had been with God, I knew that I had nothing to fear. Now I was ready to break free and begin healing.

Chapter Eleven

Once I accepted that I was forever changed with a clip in my brain, and realized that the doctors couldn't give me much guidance, I really began to live. My pace of activity quickened after the doctor appointment with the neurosurgeon in Houston. More than anything else, I wanted to get back to normal. I pushed myself. Every day I'd get out of bed and say to myself, "Okay, I'm feeling better. I think I'm stronger."

I found office space and officially opened my private practice. I was still unsure where the patients would come from, but was confident it would all work out. A friend told me about an opening for a part-time consultant at a local private school. That sounded interesting, so I interviewed with the headmaster. Although I'd never worked in such a position, it sounded like fun. I began working there two days a week in September.

My youngest daughter, Sarina, was home with me all summer. She was with me when I drove for the first time in Houston, only six weeks after my aneurysm. I was afraid to drive, but Ron was working and Sarina was too young for a license. I had to drive to the grocery and run errands. In Houston, you have to drive, as it's too far to walk most places and public transportation is difficult. I bribed Sarina to come with me on that first drive by telling her that we would go to the Container Store. It's her favorite store, as she is compulsive about organizing and likes storage boxes. By the time we arrived, my hands were shaking as I gripped the steering wheel. I was so tired when I got home from the short trip that I had to take a nap. It was difficult concentrating while driving, and the bumps still hurt my head. I was so glad that Sarina had come with me. Her strength and her confidence in me were just what I needed.

Sarina was strong in her faith that I would heal. She wouldn't talk about how afraid she was during my illness until August, nearly three months later, yet she demonstrated how to live in the moment and not feel sorry for yourself. We had moved her to Houston. She was starting a new high school, not knowing anyone. I asked her if she resented this, and her reply was one I will always cherish. She told me, "I sometimes feel lonely and sad, but I know that in the long run, this will make me stronger and better." Those were wise words from a 15-year-old girl. Sarina taught me a lot about rolling with life.

My older sister, Annie, came down to visit me on June 4. I had underestimated the importance of family in the healing process. Just having Annie here to talk with was such a comfort. She told me funny stories, sad stories. We laughed and cried. Annie took care of both of our parents before they died. Our dad died in March 2001, and mother died December 31, 2001. Annie is still grieving those deaths. She talked a lot about Mom and Dad dying, and how it was for her. It kept me connected to her and my parents, because when they died, I was in Lubbock. I was the only kid who lived far away. I felt like I'd missed some of that connection. She was very close to Mom as her main caregiver. She'd tell me little inspirational things that Mom said. That healed me so much. I have that woman's blood in me. She suffered, but was never down. If you see someone go through something and you're connected, you know that you can do it. Annie said that she knew Mom and Dad were praying for me. Hearing stories about my parents helped soothe my grief.

I told Annie about my aneurysm, which was cathartic for me. I believe that people need to talk about their experience many times in order to heal. Annie's presence healed me, as only a sister could do. I could not put a price on what it meant for me. My thinking has changed a lot because of Annie. If a family member ever became ill, I would drop everything to be with him or her.

My account of my healing process would be incomplete if I didn't mention about how I got back to my running. First of all, I must explain that running is my lifeblood. It is prayer, relaxation, and passion all rolled into an activity that I cannot imagine not doing. The doctors told me that when I started running, it would not be pleasant. They were right … it felt like shocks squirting out of my head. It made the inside of my head itch, and basically felt like my brain was hitting the side of my head. I made myself do it, slowly at first and with a very queer gait. After each run, my head would pound for a couple of hours.

At first, I walked on the treadmill at home. I alternated walking with running, doing each for a few minutes. I was terrified of going out on the streets by myself. I was scared of that feeling of my brain shutting down and of falling down. Who would know me? What would happen if it blew again and I couldn't talk? How devastating it would be for Ron. He was very nervous about my going outside, and he was happy that I was on the treadmill at home.

A close friend, Beth Dawson, was instrumental in helping me to run again. Beth came over and said, "Why don't we go over and run around Rice University? We'll go together. Have your phone number and doctor's phone number and just carry it in a packet. If something happens, I'll call." It was a great solution, as it relieved Ron's fears and helped me to feel more comfortable running outside.

We ran together three days a week. I went, no matter how bad I felt. Finally, after about three weeks, I began thinking that I really didn't need to go with Beth anymore. If the worst happened, someone would open my packet with the numbers. I carry my cell phone, so I can always call Ron. That was my ticket to freedom. I don't normally like to run with people. I have to go when they can go. I like to listen to music, and it's my meditation time. Even though Beth and I have done numerous races, I needed to know that I was still independent.

From July 16, I started walking/running 40 miles a week. I counted every walk. I took a yoga class at the community center and walked there and back. That was two miles. Summer in Houston is hot and humid, so I ran in the early morning or in the evening.

Beginning in October, I realized that it didn't hurt anymore when I ran. I started feeling like I was getting more energy. I quit walking as much and started running more. In November, I started thinking of running the Sunmart 50k (about 31 miles) in Huntsville State Park, just north of Houston. The race would be held in mid-December. My husband almost left me over my decision to run this race. Ron was so afraid that something would happen out in the middle of the woods.

"Mary, this is crazy! Why do you feel like you have to do this?"

"Because I do ... I just do!"

"But what will you do if you get sick again? It could be a long time until somebody finds you! Why do you have to take a chance?"

"I don't know, Ron, but I just have to run this race!"

Brianna is also a runner, and I asked her if she would run the race with me. She was very reluctant, because she wasn't sure that it was such a good idea either. I made a pact with her. I told her that I felt that this race was worth dying for, although I'd take precautions. I told Bri that I would stop at each 10-kilometer loop to take my blood pressure. We'd be slow. She was okay with that. She knew what could happen. I reassured her that if anything happened, she would not be at fault. I was doing the race strictly for myself. Even though I know that she was scared, she understood how important it was for me. It was a psychological passage that I had to do.

My life would not have been complete without my running that race. The only way that I could love myself was to run that race. Ron was angry, but knows me so well that he understood. I think that when you love a person, there's a level of communication between those two people that is totally not understandable to others. I know that Ron's family didn't understand my decision to run the race. I know that they were upset. Members of my family were worried. They realized how I felt about running and could see the importance for me. I think that my family's faith also grew after my illness, and they were able to trust me to make a good decision. They understood that I was no longer afraid of death; if it were God's will, it would be okay.

Early on a chilly December 13, 2003, Brianna and I set out for the park about an hour's drive from home. Just as I promised, we stopped every 10 kilometers during the race to check my blood pressure. We had so much fun. I got tired, but my endorphins must have kicked in, as everything seemed funny. Bri and I laughed and had a marvelous time. Even though I got tired, I was exhilarated.

I finished the race, and as I did, a most incredible thing happened to me. It made all of the difference in my healing. For some unknown reason, as I crossed the finish line, I began to sob...uncontrollable sobbing...from somewhere deep inside me that didn't even feel like me. Brianna instinctively knew not to enter into this private emotional release of mine. The lady who was recording my number asked me if I was okay, and I was sobbing so hard that I could only nod my head yes. I was more then okay! I was healed for the first time in seven months! I was *me* again, but better. I felt stronger at that moment then I have since in my life.

Completing that race was a much greater accomplishment than recovering from the aneurysm. Remember that running is very spiritual for me. I don't just go out there. I really listen and I pray. Even though Bri was with me, there were lots of quiet moments. It was a run of gratefulness, of celebrating my life. My body went through so much, and now I was able to be out here with all these other runners. To them, it was just another run. They were going to go as fast as they could to have a good finish. I could have come in dead last, and it would have been a victory. I don't even know what my official time was. I know that I wasn't last; it just wasn't important to me to know my standing. I was really able to live when I came back from that race. I was complete. If I had dropped dead after that, the race would have been worth it.

I think that when we have an illness, in many ways, we don't trust our bodies anymore. Our bodies have let us down. Somehow, when I crossed that finish line, I began to trust my body again, not in the old naive way that I used to, but in a new, respectful way. I respected its healing ability and its intuition. This race also taught me that healing cannot be done by what someone else thinks is appropriate. If I had listened to Ron and Brianna, I would have missed this opportunity. It is our own heart that we need to listen to, not someone else's fears.

I started working on this book during the first weeks of my recovery. I needed to do that to get this experience out of my head, to begin my healing. As I wrote about my own journey, I started thinking about all of the cancer patients that I'd met. I remembered their stories, their discoveries about life and death, and what they believed. I thought about how they felt about their illness, and how they coped with the reality of their impending death.

The chapters that follow are the stories of some of my patients. Their stories are too important not to be shared. I have changed names and minor situational issues. These patients gave me the greatest job — to be their psychotherapist while they were going through their experience with cancer. Their dying experiences ended up helping to heal me. Many of them will never know how much their lives impacted my own.

Chapter Twelve

"... and the time came when the risk it took to remain in a tightly closed bud became infinitely more painful than the risk it took to blossom."
—Anais Nin

The year was 1995. I had lived in Lubbock, Texas, for one full year. I was seeing a few patients and volunteering at hospice. I became friends with a woman named Diane Lowell, who was very involved in the Susan G. Komen Breast Cancer Foundation. Diane invited me to a wine and cheese party sponsored by the foundation. I love wine, and I thought it would be an opportunity to meet some new people, so I forced myself to go. Although I may appear outgoing, I am actually very shy, so going to a party where I don't know anyone is painful.

I met a man there who virtually changed the course of my life. I liked him the instant I met him, and I liked him more because he came up to me and started to make small talk. When you are shy, this means a lot. He was a large, soft-spoken man with gentle brown eyes. He introduced himself as Dr. Mike Ward. He told me about his practice as a cancer specialist. He asked me what I did. I told him that I was a relationship/intimacy counselor who had recently moved to Lubbock.

"Have you ever worked with cancer patients?" he asked.

"No, I haven't," I replied.

"Would you like to?"

"Well, I never thought about it."

"I'm looking for a psychotherapist who would be willing to run support groups."

"I have no experience with support groups, but I suppose that I could learn."

"Could you come by my office tomorrow for an interview?" he asked as he gave me his business card.

"Sure!" I answered, rather flippantly.

"What time can you be there?"

I hate making commitments, so I said, "How about around 2:00 p.m.?"

"Okay, then, my office at 2:00 p.m."

I left thinking I had drunk too much wine. What in the hell was I doing? I didn't know anything about cancer or cancer patients. On the way home, I stopped by the library and checked out seven books about cancer. I decided I should at least have a basic understanding of what was involved. When Ron came home, he looked at me with my pile of cancer books and asked what I was doing. I told him I had to learn everything I could about cancer before tomorrow at 2:00 p.m.

"Why?" he asked and started to laugh.

"Because I'm going to interview for a psychotherapist position with Dr. Ward."

"Mary, you don't know anything about cancer," said Ron, still somewhat laughing.

"Well, I know that and you know that, but maybe I can fool Dr. Ward."

Have you ever met someone and wondered what turn your life would have taken if you hadn't? That's how it was with Dr. Ward. The morning of my interview, I went back and forth on whether I should actually show up. He called at 10:00 a.m. to make sure that I was still coming. "Oh yes, I have it scheduled for 2:00 p.m." I felt like a liar, because I really wasn't sure that I would actually go to the interview.

I did show up, though, and quickly learned that I couldn't fool Dr. Ward about my knowledge of cancer. However, that didn't seem to matter to him. He told me that I'd be perfect for his practice. His warm, reassuring presence helped to convince me to join him. Nothing in my life would be the same after that interview. I didn't realize how much I would learn about life and myself because of this job. Eventually, it grew into something that I did full time during the next eight years in Lubbock.

My first group for Dr. Ward was to be held the following Monday. He would pay me for the groups, and any patient who wanted to see me in my private practice could make an appointment with me directly. It seemed to be a good opportunity and a chance to serve a need for his patients. I had only a weekend to prepare for the first session, and I was eager to meet my new patients.

Chapter Thirteen

Monday night I showed up early at Dr. Ward's office. The group was to begin at 6:30 p.m., but I was there by five o'clock. I met his nurses and office staff. They were excited to have this emotional support group and were supportive of me. I felt unprepared to lead a group of cancer patients. What would I say? How would they react to me? I'm healthy and young. Perhaps nobody will talk or I'll say the wrong thing.

Six people showed up for the first group. Jean and John had been married for forty-three years. John had a brain tumor. He was in stage IV, and his cancer was incurable. John was a farmer. He was thin and had a worried look on his face. He had intense blue eyes and gray hair. His wife, Jean, was a homemaker. She became the talker in the group. John listened but didn't add much to the conversation.

Emily was in her early 30s, which is young for a breast cancer patient. She was divorced, with no children. Emily had been dealing with cancer for several years and had had surgery, radiation, and chemotherapy. She was angry about her cancer, and about her life. It was unfair that she had cancer and was stuck in a group with older people. Emily felt that they have been able to live their lives, while she would die young, with her dreams unfulfilled. During one session, Emily voiced that sentiment to the group. They were empathetic, but angry. I didn't have to say much. They handled it by telling her that no matter how old you were, it was never okay to have this disease. The group must have made her feel accepted, because she returned the next week and remained a part of it.

Alana was in her mid-40s, a single mother of three young children. She had metastatic liver cancer and was orange as a carrot. She was not expected to live through the year. Compared to Emily, she didn't appear to be angry. I believe that she was too sick to be angry.

George and Ellen were married. She was in her late 50s, with short, pixie-like hair. Ellen was reserved, yet came across as a toughie (she was only five feet tall and very thin). She had a cancer of unknown primary, which means that she had cancer, but doctors were not sure where it originated. Her husband, George, was in his mid-60s, with a warm personality. He was a big teddy bear guy—overweight, with a barrel chest. He was accepting of people, and the group felt comfortable with him.

We discussed how we would run the group and decided upon the rules. It was very important to the members that what was said in the group be kept confidential. We decided to be an open group, with new patients welcomed at any time. Everyone in the group would have each other's name and phone number. This would help them so they could all support each other through painful treatments and surgeries.

Oddly enough, these patients never asked me where I trained or where I came from. They knew by my accent that I was not from West Texas, and one of them asked me if I was a gypsy (we all got a good laugh out of that), but they were very accepting of each other and me. This is not unusual in my working with cancer patients. They are, in general, the nicest and most accepting type of patient. This is part of the reason that they were so good at teaching me, and training me how to do psychotherapy with them. I never did learn how to work with cancer patients from any books that I read. I learned at the hand of the master. The patients who had cancer taught me how to listen. I realized the great healing power of listening to their fears, anger, and sadness. At the end of life, what seemed to be most important to the patients was that someone listen to them without judgment, and validate their lives.

We decided that the group would meet every Thursday from 6:30 until 7:30 p.m. For the next two years, I met these patients once a week and became part of their family. When I left Dr. Ward's practice, they followed me over to the cancer center and joined the group we started over there. We partied together, celebrating new births, remissions from cancer, last chemo treatment, and marriages. We mourned together when we lost a group member. I had a policy within the group that no event would go uncelebrated...life was too short. They loved that rule, and we all celebrated with gusto. When I left the cancer center in 2003, I grieved that group as much as I grieved the loss of my colleagues.

I went to visit Ellen in the hospital when I heard that she was very sick. She had missed the group the Thursday before, and the other patients said that she was not doing well. This visit would be my last one with her.

"How are you doing, Ellen?" I asked.

"My body is shutting down. Nothing works the way it should. You know, when you get like this, God is supposed to take you," she replied weakly.

"Are you ready for that, Ellen?" I asked.

"Oh, yes, I'm ready. I've been talking to God."

"What did God say to you?" I asked. I was curious, but very skeptical, since she was on the powerful painkiller morphine.

"He told me that I was going to be fine, that He loved me and was with me. He told me not to worry about how it would be, that I need to trust Him."

"How did God speak to you?"

"Not in words, but I hear it and understand Him."

Ellen went on to say that most of her life she had fought against death. She had always been a cautious person and afraid of getting hurt. She said, somehow, now that she was dying, she was free of fear, not afraid at all. Then she looked at me with really tired eyes, no eyelashes left or brows or hair. "Oh dear, I've been going on and on. Thank you. Thanks for listening," she said.

I was feeling guilty because I doubted that she really experienced God. As I was listening, I was thinking, "Oh, God. Do I have to listen to this? I'm tired of these stories. They should cut her morphine way down."

"Ellen," I said, "don't say thanks. This is my job, and I like visiting with you. I haven't really done much."

"Not much," she said. "You made me laugh during every one of those groups. You are so silly...I love you."

Within two days of that visit, Ellen was dead.

Doctors and scientists have told us that maybe morphine or antianxiety medications alleviate fear and it has nothing to do with a "God." I realize that this is possible, and I must be honest. I, too, was skeptical of many of the God stories. I still cannot make sense out of how patients can be so socially aware and appropriate if they are medicated to the point that they are hearing, seeing, and even feeling things. If they were so doped up that they were having what we would call hallucinations, then they wouldn't be able to talk to me in the rational manner that they did. They would not have been able to express their feelings and life stories so eloquently.

I question the medical profession and myself. Science looks for causes of why patients have these "hallucinations" and tries to explain them scientifically. Does a part of the brain shut down? Do painkillers cause patients to believe that they can sense the presence of God? I think that spending so much time and effort trying to make a scientific case for these experiences rather than listening to and accepting patients' stories is our own way of controlling the end of life.

I believe that skepticism helps us in the medical profession to emotionally disconnect from the patient. I was a nurse before I was a psychotherapist, and I will never forget the instructors telling me, "Mary Jo, you will never be a good nurse if you don't learn to disassociate from the patient." She was right. I was never a good nurse, but I make a pretty good psychotherapist (although I never did learn to disassociate very well).

John also died that year. I sat with him many times in his dying process. John was not communicative. He was a West Texas farmer who learned to work with his hands. Words were of little use to him. He showed love by what he did. He was a provider for his family. He rarely expressed how he felt about anything. When he did talk, he kept his conversations close to home. He wanted to know about the weather. That was easy. The wind was blowing and it's hot, or the wind was blowing and it's cold. John often wanted to know what I ate for breakfast or lunch. I'm not sure why it was important for him to know what I ate, but it was a way for him to make conversation.

Two days before John died, I went to see him. I arrived after lunch, and this was his naptime. He was awake, though, so I sat in the chair next to his bed. We started out with all the usual topics—the weather, food, etc. Then he blurted out something that I did not expect. "My mother came to my bed this morning," John said.

"Does she live close by?" I asked.

"No, she died eight years ago."

"What do you think about this, John?"

"Oh, I don't know. It's probably that damned medicine."

He relaxed a bit after telling me about this and asked me what I thought. "I'm not sure, but other patients have told similar stories to me. Did you feel better after your mother came, or more afraid?"

"Oh, I woke up so happy," he said.

"She must love you very much to come and see you when you're so sick," I suggested.

John smiled his crooked smile full of yellow teeth, and we were both quiet. I sat with him for a while, just being there. After a few minutes, my pager went off. I gathered my things and told John good-bye.

"Good-bye, Mary Jo. That was a good visit, wasn't it?"

"Yes," I said. "It was." In all truth, it wasn't a long, deep conversation. It was listening to someone who already had the answers. I almost screwed it up, trying to explain what was going on psychologically (as if I knew). We medical professionals often try to intellectualize things so that the patient can understand. This is a coping mechanism for us, as it helps us to separate from the patient's concerns. It also helps us to feel more in control. John died four days later and left me with more than I ever gave him.

Why are patients so reluctant to tell us health professionals about things they're seeing before they die? Are they afraid that we will judge them? Do we judge them? Are they still trying to be "a good patient"? Are we as medical professionals so caught up in the science that we are closed to experiences that have no double-blind research behind them? Do we discount the stories, blaming the medication, and then leave the room? As I read these questions, I can answer yes to several of them. How many times did I quickly exit a room after hearing one of these stories, leaving the patient feeling lonely and abandoned after telling me about a spiritual experience?

It seems logical to think that when a patient is dying or severely debilitated, he would be depressed or feeling sorry for himself. However, in my experience, many patients are more content while in the dying process than at any other time in their lives. They feel more at peace, and secure in their relationship with their God. I cannot tell you the number of patients who have told me this. It is almost as if the journeys through their illness made them understand themselves better. They are more trusting of God, or a divine fate.

I am sure there is a grieving process for what they can no longer physically do, but I am very aware of their sense of peace also. Family members will often report this peacefulness. While not every patient feels so content, a significant number of my patients did feel this way.

When I think of my time working with Dr. Ward, I think of these patients. I think of the way they died, and how they tried to share parts of their story with me. In life, everyone has something to teach. What were the lessons I learned with my first mentor and his patients?

1. I don't know anything about cancer, or how it feels to have cancer, and I should never assume that I do.

2. There is something that happens on a spiritual level that most of us in the medical community cannot see and therefore cannot validate. We must seek to understand rather than judge the patient.

3. When a patient is dying, he or she is actually clearer about other people's motives and intentions. In other words, the dying can see right through the living. That includes me as well as other health care providers. Be sincere, and do what you say you will.

Chapter Fourteen

"We are not humans having a spiritual experience on earth; we are spiritual beings having a human experience on earth."
—Dr. Wayne Dyer
The Power of Intention

I don't remember the actual date I met Dr. Melanie Oblender. A petite woman with short gray hair, she is one of those people whom you feel you have always known. The asset that most stood out with Dr. Oblender was her steel blue eyes. They shot darts if she was angry, and laughed like drunken dancers if she was happy. Dr. Oblender walks swiftly, and her mind moves in the same manner. She did not enjoy small talk; she preferred the "real stuff." She was one of the most real people I met in Lubbock, and I loved her for that. Dr. Oblender was especially fun when I could get her laughing. She had a wild laugh that took her whole body to produce. Her shoulders would move up and down with the tone of her laugh. A pediatric oncologist, Dr. Oblender became what I refer to as my second mentor (since Dr. Ward was the first oncologist that I'd worked with at the cancer center). She didn't know this would be her job (I'm sure she wouldn't have taken it), and actually I didn't either. It's only after I left Lubbock and began this book that I realized what she had taught me.

Dr. Oblender gave me two of the greatest gifts I received while being a psychotherapist for cancer patients. The first gift was her trust in me. She told me about her life. I never looked at her the same after this because she was such a remarkable woman. Her childhood could not explain how she turned out to be such a loving person. Pediatric oncology was a passion for Dr. O, as we called her. She loved kids, and they loved her. Dr. O never had any children of her own, but in effect, she was a mother to every one of her patients, and while she could intimidate adults, kids saw through her and seemed to go right for the heart. Dr. O had a tough exterior, but I'm convinced that that was to hide the largest heart I ever knew. She gave love when there was none coming back her way. I respected this about her, but mostly, I respected the way she reflected on what she was doing. Was she really making it better for the patient and family, or just putting off the inevitable?

Another example of her selflessness was in the form of a rumor about Dr. O. She was offered a raise, but told the administration that she didn't need it and that they could use it for someone else. I asked her about this, and in her own humble way, she responded, "Oh, that. That was nothing." Case closed. She didn't want to talk about it. Dr. O was very easily embarrassed. I used to love to make wild comments just to watch her face contort into redness. These were gifts, because she gave me herself…real…without the mask doctors learn to don in medical school.

The second gift Dr. O gave me was Eric. Eric was a fifteen-year-old boy of Indian descent with big, dark eyes. He had a rare blood cancer and would soon die from it. The nurses asked me to see him because he was seeing "religious symbols" that his parents did not believe in. Dr. O and I went to Eric's hospital room later that afternoon, where she introduced me. Eric loved Dr. O and would have talked to a clown if she had asked him to. After the introduction, she left the room. I wasn't sure what to say to this very ill teenager.

"Eric, what's up?" I asked.

He replied weakly, "Not much. I'm just hangin' around."

I talked to him about sports, cars, and girls. I tried to think of things he'd be interested in. He had played the trumpet before he got sick, and talked about that. He loved classical music and some blues. We talked about artists and how old they were when they first started playing their instruments.

I sat and listened for a long while, and then we started talking about his cancer. He told me he had been diagnosed two years earlier, at the age of thirteen. He said that when he first found out, he was really afraid.

"How about now? Are you afraid now?" I asked.

"No, not really, but my parents are. They think I'm going to die," he said matter-of-factly.

"What about you, Eric? Do you think you're going to die?"

"Yeah, I do."

"What makes you say that, Eric?"

"Well, something is telling me that; something inside of me."

"Like a voice?"

"Yeah, sorta. But it doesn't talk out loud. I just feel it."

"Oh, I see…hmmm…I think I've had that experience before."

"Mary Jo, can I tell you a private thing?"

"Yeah, sure."

"No, really! You can't tell any of my buddies who come here to visit." Eric had about five fifteen-year-old buddies who came to visit him after school.

"Okay, Eric. I won't tell any of your buddies who come up here," I promised him.

Eric then said, "I am seeing angels."

I wasn't surprised, because many patients reported in the past that they had seen angels. "Really, what do they look like?"

"Well, they are beautiful. They are bright and wear white robe things, or something long and drapey. They have no shoes on!" Eric seemed to be very surprised that they were barefooted.

"Are they big or little?" I asked.

"You know, just *normal*," he responded.

"Wow! Do they scare you, Eric?"

"No, they make me feel loved and warm."

"Do they talk to you?"

"No, but they do make a nice sound. It isn't really singing, but it sounds like that. It is so beautiful!"

"When do they come?"

"They usually come at night, but sometimes I see them during the day."

"How many are there, Eric?"

"I don't know, but I will count them tonight."

"Okay, you'd better remember." I was thinking that Eric must be on some medication that was causing him to hallucinate. Maybe his oxygen sats were low and he was hypoxic.

Eric closed his eyes. This conversation had exhausted him. Since I see kids only on Tuesdays and Thursdays, I told him that I would be back the day after tomorrow.

"I'm going to count the angels tonight. Don't tell my friends about them. They might laugh at me Okay?"

"Okay, don't worry Eric," I told him as I made my exit. He gave me a faint smile. He was so pale that he frightened me.

I went back to the hospital to see the pediatric patients on Thursday. Eric was not one of the kids I saw. He had died on Wednesday at 4:00 p.m. I don't know how many angels there were, but Eric does.

Eric's parents were afraid that the nurses were putting ideas of angels into Eric's mind. Aren't we all a little bit like that? I know I am. What I don't understand frightens me, and I try to think of logical reasons for stories like Eric's. Maybe there are none. Why is it that when someone is sick or dying, his or her visions are no longer trusted? Would Eric have had a better death if he could have talked about these angels to the people he loved most? Would he have left this earth feeling more supported and loved?

Dr. O used to tell me that kids were easier patients than adults to deal with when they were sick or dying. She thought it was because they were closer to their creator or soul. It seems the longer we live, the more cynical we become...the less we believe...the less faith we have in creation. Perhaps that is the gift of childhood that kept Dr. O so passionate about these little patients. They trusted more and expected less.

Lessons the Children Taught Me

1. That you have only today, so enjoy it (you can watch *Winnie the Pooh* and get your chemotherapy at the same time).

2. Let go and trust in something bigger than yourself.

3. When you are afraid, go ahead and say it. People who love you are probably scared, too, and we can all comfort each other.

4. Having cancer is not the worst thing. Not having a mommy or daddy to hold your hand is.

5. Every cancer center should have a pediatric oncology floor. The kids can model for the adult cancer patients and their families how to *live* with cancer.

Chapter Fifteen

"The world is not divine play. It is divine fate. They that are the world, man, the human person, you and I, have divine meaning. Creation happens to us, burns into us, changes us, as we tremble and swoon, we submit. We participate in Creation, we encounter the Creator, offer ourselves to Him, helpers and companions."
—Martin Buber (1878-1965)
German Jewish scholar, philosopher, and writer

I started working at the cancer center in October 1996. My interview was peculiar. They really had no psychology program in the cancer center, and had relied on the medical school's psychiatry department and private-practice therapists to help with patients who were having emotional difficulty with their cancer diagnoses. None of the people interviewing me knew what they needed with regard to psychology in the cancer center (I didn't either), except that they needed an identified psychotherapist of their own. They wanted someone they could call exclusively for their patients. I decided during the first 24 hours on the job that since no one really knew how to do this job, I would jump in and make changes as I went along. This had always worked for me in the past, and I was hoping that it would work again.

The first thing I wanted was a nice room of my own where I could see the patients. They let me use the consultation room, which was very kind of the physicians, since it had been used as a place for them to talk with patients. It later became "Mary Jo's Office." The cancer center was decorated like a sterile hotel, so I set to work, adding dim table lamps (I had to buy my own light bulbs because the bureaucracy apparently couldn't order them) and paintings from home. I put tablecloths on the tables, added a small fountain, and put out tons of potpourri. It smelled wonderful and, with the dim lighting, was relaxing from the moment you stepped into the room. I brought a portable CD player and played soft music for the patients. The room took on a life of its own...spiritual and relaxing. I started bringing fresh flowers to work. The patients lit up when they came into my office. They loved seeing color and life. Unfortunately, if the patient was neutropenic (had a low white blood cell count), he or she could not be in the room with the flowers and I would remove them. Sometimes when you are sick, you appreciate signs of life more. It seemed to make the patients less afraid, less intimidated by the whole cancer experience. I enjoyed watching them soften and become more relaxed.

The medical director of the cancer center was Dr. Evérardo (Evé) Cobos. He was a tall man of Mexican descent. He didn't walk normally; he glided. In fact, I could see him coming down the hall from a distance. Dr. Cobos had bad knees. He didn't bend them the way most people do when they walk. He didn't like to admit it, but if you walked next to him, you could hear his knees creaking. He blamed it on his shoes, but I couldn't understand how all of his shoes would make that same noise.

His face was unusual in that it looked like many ethnicities on display. His eyes were small for his rather full face. He had wide, sparse eyebrows and an Arabian nose. His ears and cheeks looked Spanish, but his mouth was Italian. I would tease Dr. Cobos about this, and he became so defensive that he brought in pictures of his mother and father. He was very proud of being an American and had immigrated to this country at the age of six.

I worked with Evé Cobos for six years. He became my third mentor and possibly the most influential. Evé Cobos loved to teach, and he taught me a lot about cancer and medicine in general, but he impacted me most with his human side. I am a psychotherapist first, and it was not what he said that made a difference in my life. It was his struggle—really every oncologist's struggle—that helped me to understand his heart and spirit. He knew that so often, no matter how hard he tried, the treatments he had available would not be enough, yet Dr. Cobos never gave up, and continually worked to encourage his patients.

This portion of the book involves Dr. Cobos's patients who came to see me or died when they were on his service. Most cancer patients don't know the human side of their doctors. This is unfortunate, because it was not Evé's "doctor side" that was his most impressive. He was certainly more comfortable in this role, but his human/soul side was his best. He hid this side of himself as much as possible, almost as a way of self-preservation. He had a temper that was alive. I never saw him get angry with a patient; he protected them at all costs. Evé was one of those people who felt anger at the injustice of "little people." He couldn't stand to see patients or people under his protection get hurt. Most of us don't like this either, but we accept that it happens...it's life. At times, it seemed to me that Evé lived some sort of fantasy in his mind. When I brought this up, he would acknowledge it, but it was fueled by the fact that Evé could not tolerate bad things happening to good people.

I admired his struggle, his sadness at death, and his optimism that the patient would live. He often seemed surprised when someone died. It wasn't that he didn't know the eventual outcome; he just believed somehow that things would turn around. His attitude fascinated me. I was often pessimistic, but compared to Dr. Cobos, I felt like I was being realistic. I was new to this work and should have felt more optimism. Since he was a very experienced doctor, I couldn't understand how he could be so hopeful for a patient's prognosis.

Evé showed me the importance of doctors' being allowed to grieve. A community such as Lubbock, Texas, enables physicians to be placed on a pedestal (actually as a wife and observer, I think the physician, wife, and children are all on that pedestal). What happens when we are just human? Where do we go? Whom do we confide in? No matter where others or a community might place you, at night you have to sleep with your own heart and thoughts. No matter where you are in someone else's eyes, you have to be clear in your own. How can the health care staff ever support patients in their grief if they have no support in their own?

Working with Dr. Cobos afforded me the opportunity to work with a variety of patients, many with advanced disease. The cancer center was affiliated with the County Hospital. It seemed that we had more patients from isolated, small, West Texas towns. Many of our patients didn't have health insurance, and therefore they ignored their illness and tried to "doctor" themselves before coming for help. Most were anxious and fearful. They were easily intimidated by the medical staff and didn't understand what their illness was or the course of treatment they would have to endure.

I remember one woman vividly. She had come to our center for "breast pain." When Dr. Cobos saw her (which wasn't easy because of her fear of showing anyone, especially a doctor), her breast looked like a volcano. If I hadn't seen it, I would not have believed what untreated breast cancer could look like. It was actually black and looked jagged and raw. You could not tell her that she had cancer; she was so terrified of the disease that she ignored it.

Some health professionals would say patients like Rosita are in denial. We would make a mistake if we labeled her that way. She wasn't in denial. She knew full well that she had cancer. She was private and wanted to tell herself what it was. She came for every treatment, and actually ended up tolerating the whole cancer experience quite well. Rosita taught me so much about how important it is for each of us to reframe our illness so that our heart and soul can still live in a very ill body. Even though Rosita was still terrified, what she told herself about her disease made it appear to her as if there was still hope.

The cancer center was a teaching hospital, so each Wednesday, we all "rounded on the floor" as a team to discuss each patient. The team included a dietician, a pharmacist, nurses, a social worker, a reverend, the intern, residents, the attending physician, and me. We would walk from room to room, crowding around the patient's bed. The attending physician would talk to the patient and tell him or her the treatment plan. It most likely was a bit intimidating for the patient, although most of them acted like they didn't mind. However, they would crack jokes, and you could sense their anxiety about so many people coming to visit.

It was during one of those Wednesday rounds that I met Bert. He was a construction worker, a big guy who was in his early 40s. He looked uncomfortable in the somewhat feminine hospital gown. He was having difficulty breathing and looked very anxious. Bert had acute leukemia which was in an advanced stage. He had felt more tired than usual for the past two months. His shortness of breath is what concerned him enough to come to the hospital.

Bert had a bad type of cancer, but his family life was in worse shape than his body. He lived with his wife and child, but basically, he was alone. He received little emotional support from his family. Bert's wife loved drama, and the cancer center afforded her the perfect stage. Evidently, she didn't like Bert getting the attention. She enjoyed causing a commotion on the floor, and several times screamed at nurses and other employees. Bert was too sick to control anyone or anything except his own next breath, but I could see his dismay at her antics. It was clear that Bert's home life was totally chaotic, and his family only added to the stress of his illness.

We forget that when people get sick and are in the hospital, they don't bring just themselves with their illness. They bring their whole family. Hospital employees don't care just for the patient, they care for everyone in the family. Every hospital employee with direct patient contact impacts the family. If a family member is having emotional problems, we deal with that, too. I was not prepared for that aspect of oncology counseling. The patient seems to respond better to treatment if we can stabilize the family.

Bert deteriorated quickly after his initial diagnosis. Late one afternoon, I stopped by to visit him. With his oxygen mask on, he asked me to get his trousers from the closet. I wondered if he was going to run away from all of this. (He wouldn't have made it out of the bed. He was close to death.) I brought the slacks to him, and he fumbled for his wallet. He was shaky and weak. This took several minutes. When I offered to help, he *DEMANDED* that he wanted to do it on his own. Bert's shaking hands opened the wallet and took out a small piece of paper from a fortune cookie he had saved. "Read it to me," he said in a voice muffled by the oxygen mask.

"It says, 'Good Things Will Be Coming Your Way."

He smiled while I read the fortune. "See, Mary Jo, I will get better!" he said.

"Yes, you will! One way or another, things will improve," I responded.

Bert was satisfied with my response. He relaxed, although he was sweating profusely. His rapid, labored breathing continued. I was thinking that it would be gracious for God to take him at this moment. He was working so hard to breathe, it was painful for me to watch. His wife had signed a DNR (do not resuscitate) form, so he would not be placed on a respirator. I could tell that Bert was terrified to die, yet at that moment, he seemed more at peace.

Bert did die later that night. It happened very quickly … he bled and went into heart failure. I will never forget the way that he frantically searched for that fortune. It was touching how something so simple could offer him peace and reassurance in the last hours of his life.

He never got to communicate with his family about their lives. It felt like years of unsaid feelings when they were together. Bert taught me how a patient's family can impact his treatment and healing. I felt like I failed him in regard to his being able to mend old wounds before he died. I kept thinking that his family would be in to help comfort him, but they stayed away. He was alone in his life and at the time of his death. I became much more sensitive to the patient's family after Bert. I learned to include the family right away with the emotional treatment plan. I also found that talking with them separately from the patient allowed the family to ask questions and to voice their fears without worrying about upsetting the patient.

The patient that touched me the deepest was 49-year-old Angela. She had been a patient under the care of Dr Cobos for a long while before I met her. She was small and fair with big blue eyes. Angela had survived nine years with colon cancer. I saw more chemotherapy go into Angela's body than I could have imagined. She would have it no other way. Angela identified herself as a mother. She had one son, who was eleven at the time of her death. To Angela, death meant abandonment of her son. This was unacceptable to her, and she fought with sheer willpower and good medical care to keep going.

She wasn't religious, but talked about spiritual concepts that gave her strength. Angela believed that God always has a reason for everything. She felt that nothing happens randomly. Angela had been abused as a child, and this turned her into a very guarded person. She was suspicious of others and controlling about her treatment. Angela would request more chemo even when the doctors told her this was not advised. She was also very particular about where things belonged in her hospital room. Angela had things placed just where she wanted them. We began to ask her "Where does this belong?" It was her way of feeling in control of something since she had so little control of her own body.

Angela was in and out of consciousness for the last week of her life. It was difficult for all of the nursing staff, since they had known and loved her for nine years. I would walk into her room and hug her, talk to her, and stare at her lifeless form. Angela's husband and child lay on the bed with her. Her child would softly rub the top of her bald head.

One day I came in and Angela was alone. She looked dead—cold and devoid of any life. I greeted her and started making small talk. All of a sudden, she breathed deep, half opened one of her eyes, and said, with a hint of animation that I hadn't heard all week, "Can you see them?" I almost fainted...I was scared and shocked. I did not expect her to respond.

"No," I replied shakily. "No, Angela, I cannot see them."

"They're all over. Look! They are beautiful!"

"Angela, I can't see them," I responded, feeling almost panicked.

"Oh," she said, and then relaxed and quit talking.

I was freaking out! I tried to wake her again, but she didn't respond.

I walked quickly from Angela's room and ran into a resident. I told him what had transpired, and he said he would go check out her "levels." I assumed that he thought that she had had too much morphine, or perhaps another blood chemistry level was off, which could account for her seeing things. He probably thought that *I* was hallucinating. Believe me, I questioned it, too. Angela died a few days later, never regaining consciousness.

Afterward, I talked with Dr. Cobos about the experience. I got the answer that I thought he would give. In a way, this comforted me. He thought that perhaps I had imagined some of it, since I was emotionally close to her. Dr. Cobos said that I may have projected my own wishes onto her, or perhaps she was just hallucinating. At the time, that made sense to me. I thought about this experience a lot. What happened to Angela? Was it the medicine? Was it lack of oxygen? If it was that, why were her sentences stated so clearly? She wasn't religious, so what was Angela seeing that I could not? Whatever it was, it gave her peace and joy. Her right eye opened, and for a short time I saw life in her. Before my accident, I thought surely this had a medical or psychological answer. Now, I am quite convinced it has a spiritual answer.

Angela was the patient who started my spiritual quest at the cancer center. I questioned what I thought, and I began to read more and more about death and dying. Angela dealt with her disease by getting out of herself. She invested in her family and others to help take her mind off her own illness. This offered Angela a reason to live, to persevere even when she was nauseated and weak.

When I reflect back on the impact that she had on my life, I realize that it wasn't her cancer or her fight for life. It was more that Angela was too real to me. I identified with her emotionally. I didn't have a place or compartment for her in my mind, where I could keep her safely rationalized away. I have read about this happening, how some patients just affect you differently. When Angela laughed or cried, I could feel her emotions in myself. I experienced a heightened sense of empathy for her. I'm not sure I understand it now, but I'm quite sure that it wasn't healthy for either of us. I was no longer objective about her. I became anxious when she became sicker. When she was dying, I felt like a part of me was dying, too. Angela forced me to consider my own death.

Healing Lessons Inspired by Dr. Cobos's Patients

1. To find your purpose during times of illness, give your life away to others. On your worst days, focus on something you can do for someone else. This will prevent your feeling like a burden to your family. No matter how small, keep giving like Angela did. Angela served her family even on her sickest days. She was terribly ill on Valentine's Day, but got dressed and put makeup on to take decorated cookies to her son's class. Angela knew how important it was for her son that she bring the cookies, and she didn't want to let him down.

2. When you are ill with cancer or any other disease, talk to yourself as if you are healed. Rosita knew she had cancer, but she

would not use that word. She called it something else, and went through the cancer treatment to help heal it. Many people have difficulty with this. Psychologists call it denial and say it's pathological. I say, "Let's not judge what helps another heal." My job at the cancer center was to embrace the patients and empower them to heal their hearts and souls. I am not smart enough to tell people that their methods are not okay and that they should use mine; are you?

3. The importance of human touch can never be underestimated. Even at times of terminal illness and actual dying, the body responds to being touched in a loving and gentle way. Cancer patients, indeed, anyone suffering, often feel alone and isolated from the ones they love. They are not comfortable telling their doctors about sex-related issues they struggle with. We all need to touch and feel loved by our partners. Sex is important for health also; it contributes to stimulating T-cell activity, which supports the immune system. One of my cancer patients told me that after radiation of the vulva and painful sexual intercourse, her OB/GYN doctor told her that she should be grateful to be alive and to forget about sex. This is terrible advice from anyone, but your own OB/GYN doctor? Shame on him! Sexuality between two people is sacred, the highest level of intimacy. It's a spiritual form of expressing yourself intimately to another human being. Of course we need that to heal. I needed that to heal, and to feel feminine and healthy again.

4. Stay away from thoughts and people who weaken you. Embrace the people and readings that make you feel stronger. Bert was dying, and he knew what he needed to hear to give him strength. If I had tried to bring in his family for a "last powwow," that would have been a disaster for Bert. He understood that the communication with his family would weaken him, and he wasn't strong enough to deal with it.

5. If listening is the key to healing, then the best healers in the hospital are the housekeepers. Day after day, they clean the patients'

rooms. They talk with them and listen to them. In the Bone Marrow Unit, the patients would be there for a month at a time. Many continued correspondence with the housekeepers after their discharge. The housekeepers are unassuming and nonthreatening to the patients. They take the patients where they are that day. When I had my aneurysm, the housekeepers were the best psychotherapists. They reassured me every day, and actually listened as they mopped my floor and cleaned my mess. I owe them so much gratitude for their help and concern. Many times housekeepers don't speak English; however, listening is not about talking. They are able to demonstrate compassion and hope by a pat on the arm and soft words. Everyone can feel the comfort of being called "mi niña," or "my child," when ill. I believe that every health care professional in the hospital should express his or her thanks to these hardworking, underappreciated workers. Their job is considered menial. This is most ironic.

Chapter Sixteen

"To believe in God for me is to feel that there is a God, not a dead one, or a stuffed one, but a living one with irresistible force urging us toward more loving."
—Vincent van Gogh (1853-1890)

I left the cancer center the last day of February 2003. I left with a heavy heart, knowing that I was leaving patients I would never see again. I look back and cannot believe how those six years at the cancer center had changed me. I had seen more suffering and celebration than at any other place I had ever worked. I had my aneurysm on April 19, 2003, only one and a half months after I left my job. Was that fate? Did I have that job to prepare me for my own crisis? Was there a sense in my own soul that this would happen? These are questions that I often ask myself.

I'm not sure why God chose the order for working with cancer patients and then the aneurysm, because I could have been so much more helpful to my patients had my illness happened first. But because it happened the way it did, it's really *my* blessing. In one sense now, it seems perfectly planned. If I hadn't worked with cancer patients, I would not have been as effective at healing my heart and soul after the surgery. The surgery was a small part of my cerebral aneurysm. The healing part took years and lots of reflection.

Now I realize that I have to use my blessing. I can't go back to the cancer center. Those people are gone now. I was given a second chance, and that puts more responsibility on me to give and to love others. I still question that perhaps it would have been better if God had put my work and illness in a different order. I regret many of the thoughts and ideas I had along the way. Maybe the reason He did that is because He didn't think that I would learn from the aneurysm. He realized that the patients had already taught me the lessons, and the experience I had only deepened it. Before, I probably wouldn't have been as committed. The whole process deepened my faith that there is a God, that there *is* so much more, and that He does have your best interests at heart. There is a plan for your life. You might feel that you're changing the plan or creating parts of it. That's where free choice comes in. Maybe you can do a little bit, but ultimately it's planned for you. I have a trust in God that I couldn't have gotten any other way. I admire anybody who has the trust that I have without having had to go through what I did.

My patients have told me that they just leave it up to God; they trust Him so much. I used to never be able to say that. I never felt brave enough to trust God to the extent that I would allow His will to be done, but that is the very thing that healed me. My experience taught me that submitting is realizing that I really don't have control. By resolving the conflict between the illusion of control and submitting to another power, I learned that trusting God makes me very powerful.

When it was apparent that cancer patients were dying, it was not a morbid thing. It was a celebration. I felt so fortunate to be with them at that time. I witnessed their healing. They were healed in the sense that they had a deeper understanding of life. Something or someone was already talking to them on another level. They weren't the same; many patients were calmer. I could see that they were able to let go. They were at peace. The families had a difficult time saying good-bye. I know that a lot of times we pray for people to physically heal, yet the loved one dies. Families may believe that God didn't answer their prayers since the patient died. But I witnessed many times that same loved one healed in his or her heart and soul, and I believe that prayer helped ease the way.

People have asked me many times if I have become religious. I was a double major in theology and psychology. I respect all religions. I respect God, or Creator, if you will. I have become much more spiritual. I attend a Roman Catholic Church because there's a familiarity with it that comforts me. I believe that I have become much more spiritual than religious. I have complete faith in God, and believe there is another world. Whether you call that heaven or not, I will leave it for you to interpret.

People ask if there's a hell. I don't know. I didn't see any evidence of it. Were there angels? I think perhaps there were, but I don't have enough of the facts to know. I wasn't there long enough, but I was there long enough that it changed my life. That's how powerful it was.

When I was in that brilliant pink room, I was naked … only my essence was of importance to God. I don't remember being aware of the rest of my body with me. I could see, but I didn't use my eyes in the same way. They were more to see the beauty, which was breathtaking. I felt knowingness, and God's message came through my skin, or through the essence of me. I didn't see God, but I knew I was with Him. It's hard to use words to explain the experience, because we are limited in our understanding. Things have to be tangible, or seen, here. When I was with God, these tangible or concrete senses were of no importance. When I was born, I came to this earth naked, just me. That is how I went back to God. I was naked, just me.

I was held by a loving Creator. He was fatherly in the sense that I felt very safe and protected. The room was full of an incredible sensation of love and peace. It was so beautiful. I love life. For the most part, I'm in love with life, yet I would have given anything to stay in that place with God. I'm an intellectual person—I know that my story sounds corny. I wouldn't have believed it myself if I hadn't experienced it. People have suggested that my near-death experience was caused by medication. I was never given any painkillers or medication that would have produced hallucinations. Since I'm a runner, I've experienced endorphins. The radiant room was nothing like the runner's high that I have felt many times.

A few months after my experience, I asked Ron if he'd been able to tell that I'd left the room. "You were in and out of awareness while the doctors were talking," he said. "You looked peaceful. Usually when I'd say, 'Mary!' you'd wake and say, 'Yeah, I'm here.' But one time you didn't wake up. That really scared me. I called you again, 'Mary, Mary! Still with us?' Finally you opened your eyes and asked me to hold your head."

Ron thought that my central nervous system (CNS) must have been depressed, because I was so calm.

"But if my CNS was depressed, wouldn't I have been more groggy?

"Was I depressed?" I asked Ron.

"No. It wasn't depression. You were eager to do what the doctors said. You wanted to get up and move. It was just that you were so calm. It freaked me out because you weren't grabbing onto me, crying, 'You've got to help me!' Your head hurt, and you asked me to hold your head, but I never saw you scared," said Ron.

"Mary, if you went to be with God, and you knew that you were going to live, a normal person would be elated about getting another chance to live. I don't understand why you were so unhappy to wake up back on earth."

"I think this is what we humans don't understand. It is such peace. All I could think of when I opened my eyes and saw that I was back on earth again was 'Oh, shit! Oh, my God! You've got to be kidding!' I've got to wake up to this now. I knew that I was going to have surgery. I knew that I wasn't going to die during the operation. I was pretty sure that I was going to be okay."

I couldn't imagine that God would say, "You could love more," and then take everything away, although He could have … He can do anything He wants. The way He said it was, "You need to shape up. You need to get your act together." It almost felt like God was telling me, "I gave you so much. You're not using it enough." I took those words very literally and complained that I'd given so much already. The cancer center paid me $600 a month to see their cancer patients. I was at the cancer center three days a week, so I felt that I'd devoted quite enough of my life to caring for others. It was a shock to learn that I had more loving and giving to do in my life.

In a sense, I did die with my aneurysm. I died to old thoughts and judgments that were not helpful in my life. I had made judgments about people and situations that were not true. I was becoming more and more skeptical of a God or afterlife. With my near-death experience, I learned to have more faith in the things I can't see or touch. I accept that there is a God. Rather than close myself to possibilities, I've become open to whatever He wants of me.

I had my own resurrection. I don't look any different, but I have changed so much. I loved myself then but admire myself now. I like my choices, how I look at life. I'm grateful for the new perspective. I have a lot more understanding, and it has taken away most of my anxieties. I'm no longer preoccupied with becoming ill or dying. I have very little fear. I like who I am now much better.

I realize that seeing angels or having near-death experiences does not happen to everyone. Many people get close to death and just pass. Many fight and struggle and then die without expressing anything. Some people look like the painting *The Scream* before they die. I remember one man who died, and he scared me because he looked exactly like the painting. I cannot explain this, and I have no desire to try anymore.

Where am I now, after three years? I work in a Houston, Texas, hospital. I help patients continue their journeys through near death and dying. I hear their stories, and learn what patients experience during that time. It is still as fascinating as the first story I ever heard, but I am different now. I listen more. I smile with them. I release them to what they see. I no longer ask the physician what medications they are on. I include their family more, and try to support their whole experience. I am in a sense "healed" from my own pathology of needing a reason or a scientific explanation for what I experienced.

I also have a private practice, where I specialize in treating sexual problems and relationship issues, and I evaluate patients to determine their psychological readiness for weight-reduction surgery. Last year, after seeing a number of adolescent girls and young women with body image issues, I decided to produce a TV show on a local cable access channel. Called "The Mary Jo Show," it airs bimonthly and features interviews with area teens. We discuss many topics, with the goal of educating and empowering them.

I'm still running 40-50 miles a week. Weight lifting has been significantly modified. I no longer lift more than ten pounds over my head. (My husband is probably hoping that one of those weights will hit my head, to knock some sense into it!)

Motivational speaking has also begun to take up a lot of my time. I speak to community groups about topics from spirituality to sexuality to coping with illness. I am also a volunteer lobbyist for the American Cancer Society, and have lobbied at the state government for increased cancer funding.

I hope that by telling my story, it will inspire you to stop and reflect on your own beliefs. What is God to you? What are your fears or concerns about death? What is your purpose here? What else can you give before you leave this earth? What are you giving right now that makes you happy?

If you are ill, I would like to offer you hope. You are ongoing. You are much more than you can imagine, and so is the universe. Your life here is only one small chapter of a book. You have sent ripples out which will continue to widen and grow. Suffering opens the way to examining our old thoughts and prejudices that hold us back. The more we let go of these, the more open we become to being healed. A near-death experience brings you these insights sooner…you have new priorities and see life differently. But something happens to all of us eventually. An event occurs in life that becomes a catalyst for change. For me, that catalyst was a brain aneurysm. For you it may be something different, but if you stay open and have faith, you will be guided.

If you are in the process of your own death, or going through the death process with a loved one, have faith in the concept that even at this dark, bleak time, healing is happening. Most of us have to come very close to death to realize that it is within this dying that we are actually healing. It was when I was dying in my physical sense that I was healing in my spiritual/emotional sense. Our physical bodies are limited; our spiritual/emotional sense is limitless.

To all the medical professionals I worked with, I would like to say "thank you." Thank you for your dedication and caring for your patients and me. My neurosurgeon was, without a doubt, the perfect doctor for me. He let me ask questions and treated me with great respect. He understood when I told him I had to move and exercise and get back to my life. He never said no. Instead, he suggested ways to ease back into my very active life. Some of the time I listened to him, and I regretted the times I did not, because I would get a whopping headache. All of my physicians were incredible, and I owe them many thanks.

I would like to challenge everyone reading this book to try and listen more. How did we forget that we work for the patient? The patient doesn't work for the doctor, health care professionals, or even his or her family. The patient is the boss. We are supposed to guide patients, and help heal them. Let the dying patient be heard. I think he or she has a lot to say if we remain nonjudgmental and curious. I think the way we hand a patient back to God makes a big statement. Did we love him or her enough to show kindness, empathy, and respect? Did we consider the patient's family and how instrumental they would be in helping their family member die? Can we do better?

To my God, I would like to say "Thank You" for the blessing of my own illness and for allowing me to be present when patients were dying. I did not realize at the time what a wonderful gift You had given me. I remember what You told me in that brilliant pink room the short while that I was with You: "Love others the way you feel love here." If this book is able to translate any of God's love for you, then maybe I am making good on that one simple, but very difficult, request.

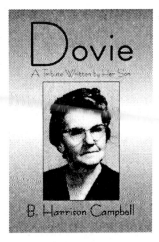